Origins and Development
of Medical Imaging

Medical Humanities Series

Theodore R. LeBlang, *Editor*
Glen W. Davidson, *Senior Consulting Editor*

The Medical Humanities Series is sponsored by the Department of Medical Humanities at Southern Illinois University School of Medicine in Springfield. The series is devoted to publication of original materials that contribute insights from the humanities on medicine, including medical education, clinical practice, and health care delivery.

The Editor encourages submission of manuscripts in the areas of anthropology, ethics, health policy, history, law, literature, philosophy, psychosocial care, religious studies, and the visual arts.

Inquiries should be directed to the Editor, Department of Medical Humanities-1113, Southern Illinois University School of Medicine, P.O. Box 19230, Springfield, IL 62794-1113.

Origins and Development of Medical Imaging

T. DOBY

G. ALKER

SOUTHERN ILLINOIS UNIVERSITY PRESS
Carbondale and Edwardsville

Library of Congress Cataloging-in-Publication Data
Doby, T. (Tibor)
Origins and development of medical imaging / T. Doby and G. Alker.
    p.   cm. — (Medical humanities series)
    Includes bibliographical references and index.
    1. Diagnostic imaging—History. 2. Radiography, Medical—
History.
    I. Alker, George J. II. Title. III. Series
       [DNLM: 1. Diagnostic Imaging—history.   WN 11.1 D635o
    1996]
    RC78.7.D53D63   1997
    616.07'54'09—dc20
    DNLM/DLC
    for Library of Congress   96-8134
    ISBN 0-8093-2010-X (alk. paper)   CIP

Contents

Plates

Preface

AT A RECENT INTERNATIONAL MEDICAL MEETING, a professor of radiology showed an aerial view of new additions to a West European hospital, pointing out that the imaging department took the largest space, outstripping by far the additions of all other departments collectively. He followed his demonstration by telling of his last encounter with a sales representative for new diagnostic equipment, in which he was presented with a sophisticated innovation unheard of previously, prompting him to exclaim in desperation: "Stop it, please stop it. We cannot follow the rapid changes any more in such a short time." The professor's plea will not be heeded, however; technology will proceed further and further.

This onslaught of novelties almost forces us to pause for a moment to consider how far we have come, and from where and under what kinds of circumstances. Seeing the inside of the human body has been delayed for a very long time. Our medical knowledge was lopsided, even blindfolded, because for thousands of years theory worked, at best, without the sobering insight into the human body. Only relatively recently have we been able to look into organs and the whole body—with spectacular results. This book traces the development of our ability to see the inside of the body—meanwhile, of course, not forgetting the importance of the invisible in medicine.

We give a sweeping survey of the forward leaps of medical science gained by looking and seeing. With such an enormous program we faced two possibilities: either to publish a series of volumes by numerous authors to unravel all the particulars that such a vast territory of knowledge requires or to try to combine the principal data in a concise space under a unifying style to give a picture of the whole. And the latter is exactly what we attempt to undertake. The evolution of *seeing* in medical history is demonstrated as we cast our eyes toward the present-day achievements. Only by looking at past events with an understanding of the difficulties our predecessors had to face can we hope that our efforts will be understood and appreciated in the future.

Inevitably we had to omit details that might have been interesting, but the notes section nevertheless gives the reader information on where to search for more data. Readers seeking specific information on the most recent technology or on experimental efforts to advance our imaging potentials must consult other works or the excellent journals, yearbooks, and annals published by professional societies. This book is about the great leaps of imagination and the achievements that brought us to the computer age—and who knows where beyond?

Acknowledgments

WE CANNOT FORGET to say many thanks to those who have read our manuscript and made valuable suggestions, including J. Cameron (professor of physics, University of Wisconsin), J. L. Doppman (professor of diagnostic radiology, Georgetown University), J. H. Scatliff (professor of diagnostic radiology, University of North Carolina), and P. Schimert (clinical professor of internal medicine, Abraham Lincoln School of Medicine, University of Illinois at Chicago). We found much-appreciated help in finding books and doing research in the vast resources of the Yale University Medical Historical Library with the assistance and guidance of librarian Frank Gyorgyei. Illustrations were taken from acknowledged historical books and from our radiology departments with the help of Dr. Steve Austin; Lt. Colonel E. B. Severson contributed toward the photographic work. Judy Barrington from the Audio-Visual Department of the Maine Medical Center (Portland, Maine) was also helpful. Mary Ellen McElligott of Southern Illinois University School of Medicine is due special thanks for the preparation of the manuscript with many important observations and arrangement of illustrations and proofreading. Ruth Kissell, our copyeditor, was also helpful with editorial remarks. Joan Notar performed well-appreciated secretarial work.

Last but not least, our thanks go to our wives, Anny Doby and June Alker, without whose patience, endurance, and friendly criticism this book would not have been finished. And for the future: We will be grateful for any suggestions or opinions reflecting the view of the reader.

1

Early Beliefs about the Human Body, 4000–300 B.C.

HORROR OF the dead, superstition, and oppressive decrees prevented our ancestors from taking a look at the inside of the human body. But do those forebears deserve to be ridiculed just because they did not practice the golden rules of scientific methodology? The first known homo sapiens more than thirty thousand years ago had the same skull capacity as we do, consequently the same brain weight and number of nerve cells.[1] And they had the same "brain hardware," lacking only our accumulated experience of thousands of years.

In ancient times disease was thought to originate from evil spirits sent as punishment by the gods; to dismember or open a dead body would evoke the vengeance of the spirits. These people explained events through similarity, analogy, and unrelated things happening synchronously. When they established what they thought were cause-and-effect relationships, they sanctioned and perpetuated them as ritual.

Prehistoric people did have considerable contact with animals, however. Hunting and butchering gave them the opportunity to look inside animal bodies. But they lived in constant battle for survival; most people died in their twenties, thus deprived of time and opportunity for more thinking, accumulation of experience, and a desire to compare. A few valid observations were submerged into a sea of false beliefs.

Egypt

It is misleading to characterize Egyptian medicine under a simple heading, for the span of years between 4000 and 300 B.C. represented decline as well as progress. The development of medical knowledge was restricted by lack of communication, fear of reprimand from the ruling classes, and the people's vision of life, death, and gods. Superstition, belief in magic, and fear of the gods limited their knowledge of the human body.[2]

The Egyptians derived flashes of insight from random deductions. For example, when they discovered that the urine of pregnant women made plants grow, they developed a pregnancy test, but they did not apply that insight beyond pregnancy. The Egyptians never transferred the observation to other areas or pursue it in detail.

The Egyptians listed the main arteries and veins, and they recognized the heart as the center of blood supply. Some described the brain with its convolutions and the meninges as the site of mental functions, but others thought the heart and intestines were the seat of the mind.[3] The uterus was thought to have two horns, and the heart and trachea were thought to be identical with those of cattle.[4] Anatomical concepts were derived from animal models. The Egyptians' clinical observations and logic were excellent. Having seen the abundant number of parasites causing disease, they deduced that even those diseases where inspection did not reveal parasites must have been caused by worms not visible to the naked eye—a preview of microscopy. The Egyptians even had an "Office for Measuring Drugs." They gave proper instructions for the treatment of fractures, dislocations, and wounds.[5]

One would think that the priests entrusted with the care of patients would have a reasonable knowledge of human anatomy and pathology since they carried out embalmments. It appears that they were more concerned with ritual than with investigation of the human body.[6] Imagination triggered by religious teachings outweighed experience. Observations were mixed with superstitions.

Their prescriptions included blood, fat, brain, and fecal material of donkeys, lizards, lions, cats, lice, and other creatures. Despite all this, the Egyptians described symptoms of apoplexy, plague, rheumatism, tumors, and skin and venereal diseases.

To summarize, although Egyptian medicine had a profound influence on Greek and therefore our own medicine, it was actually a mixture of the rational and the irrational.

The Middle East

In Mesopotamia, astronomy was developed to an extensive degree and it influenced all facets of Sumerian, Akkadian, and Babylonian-Assyrian life. The reason was water. The flooding and receding of the rivers and the blooming and withering of plants paralleled the changes in the seasons. Even certain diseases were seasonal as was the changing position of the sun and the stars. Everything seemed to be linked with the heavenly bodies.

The priests who were well versed in mathematical calculations and astronomical observations interpreted symptoms of diseases and their cure. But the supposed interplay of heavenly bodies and medicine went so far that, for example, certain medicinal herbs had to be collected in moonlight; otherwise, they would not be effective.[7] In animal sacrifices, the priests first looked at the liver, believing that its form or irregularities would provide the clue for diagnosis and prognosis because the liver was supposed to be the center of blood supply and the seat of the soul. Although the clay models of livers used to teach the new generation of soothsayers about their art represented a fair depiction of the human liver, contact with corpses was held to be "unclean"and dissection was discouraged. The Mesopotamians developed instruments for surgical procedures—although they regarded surgical intervention as dangerous to patient and surgeon alike. The code of Hammurabi declared: "If a physician shall produce on anyone a wound with a bronze knife and cure him . . . he shall receive ten shekels of silver . . . [but if he will] kill him, or shall open an abscess . . . and destroy the eye, his hands shall be cut off."[8]

Few "books" (clay tablets with cuneiform inscriptions) dealing with medicine failed to repeat the magical lore common to those times. History generally records widely accepted explanations and ignores differing opinions. So the rational approach was superseded by the accepted magical explanations.

The holy scripts of the Jews reveal a great understanding of human health and disease. Jewish sanitary regulations of home and community gain our unrestricted praise. Extensive literature points to their observations on leprosy and their recognition of animal vectors of disease in such epidemics as bubonic plague.[9] For example, the Hebrew scriptures state that mice "died and marred the land" in an epidemic.[10] But the restrictions against dissection of human bodies hampered a deeper understanding. According to the scholar Rosner: "Only God could heal sickness. In Israel there were only 'helpers' who treated patients. Those physicians who called themselves *rofe* (healer) were foreigners as a rule, and are mentioned in a derogatory fashion. . . . The main emphasis is not put on therapy, but on preventive medicine and physical and mental hygiene, as applied to the individual, the family, the people and society in general."[11]

Ancient India and China
India and China have special fascination for those who are interested in occult philosophy and the practices of Yoga and Zen, though Western disciples of these Oriental doctrines do not take into account the slowing and numbing effects of a hot climate and drugs.

Teaching of anatomy in ancient India—and Susruta, the leading physician of the sixth century, stressed its importance—was performed in a unique way: According to religious law, the organs had to be put into a bag and allowed to rot in a river for seven days; they were then dissected without using a knife.[12] Prognostics were influenced by incidental occurrences: If the messenger sent to the physician was wearing white, the interpretation was favorable. If the physician on the way to the patient met a virgin, or two (not one) Brahmins, the outlook was also favorable.[13] Despite solid surgical methods—including rhinoplasty, favorable wound dressing, good suture materials, a variety of well-designed surgical instruments, and needles—the lack of proper pathological proof prevented Indians from developing full-fledged scientific medicine.

The importance of dissections and surgical skills so ably promoted by Susruta had declined after the introduction of Buddhism in the fourth century.[14]

In ancient China, anatomy was not investigated because Confucius thought that the human body was sacred and in death should not be touched. As a result, surgery did not develop; medical concepts were bound by rigid adherence to tradition and application of the principles of Yang (representing the concepts of light, strength, and energy) and Yin (representing the concepts of darkness, weakness, and rest). Such teachings as "the 'this' is also 'that'"[15] did not lead to any tangible notion in medicine. Such doctrines as the "intelligent soul" having its seat in the liver and the "living soul" in the middle of the breast (thorax) were believed century after century.

The inoculation for smallpox prevention by taking a crust from the pustule, pulverizing it, and introducing the powder into the nostril by blowing it through a bamboo tube, gains our admiration.[16] However, defense mechanism by humors or organs was not explored; thus, this marvelous observation of the body's immune system did not trigger further development.[17]

Greece
Greece—a latecomer after Egypt, Mesopotamia, and the Orient—incorporated scientific notions from each culture. There was, however, a great difference between teacher and pupil. The Greeks lacked a centralized state: each city-state had a separate government, different customs, and its own gods. Certainly the stronger cities sought to dominate the weaker ones, but geography curbed aggrandizement. The people were scattered in valleys and islands, protected by seas and mountains. Armies could not impose dominance easily over all Greek-speaking people as they could on the plains of Egypt and Mesopotamia. The city-states flourished separately and conducted their own affairs. To avoid threats from foreign nations, or for profit, they sometimes joined their efforts in loose temporary alliances such as the twelve cities of Ionia (Dodecapolis) in Asia Minor and the six cities of the Dorians around Rhodes (Hexapolis).[18] The development of representative government and free elections among the Greeks and their bent

toward unrestricted criticism created a climate for free inquiry. The same critical freedom was obvious in their religious life: no strict dogmas were laid down. Although the Greeks acted not infrequently on the guidance of their gods as interpreted by their priests, the priests themselves held office temporarily, for the priestly office was passed from citizen to citizen.

Critical freedom in governmental and religious matters was reflected in their views about nature as well. The origins of the universe, as well as the sun, the moon, the stars, and their relation to the earth, were discussed in various cities in various ways. Clashing opinions were weighed against credibility or logic or reasoning, not religious, philosophical, or political dictates. Life and death, health and disease were examined for their natural appearance or reasonable relationships to each other—as far as could be seen—but not as a consequence of supernatural forces.

Philosophers of different cities gave emphasis to different things: In Miletos, Democritus (460–370 B.C.) taught the first version of atomic theory, saying that everything was made up of atoms, some larger, some smaller. Even the "soul," he said, was nothing but a combination of the finest fire atoms. He stated that the perception of our senses was also based on the movement of atoms; if biochemically active molecules are substituted for atoms, the concept seems quite modern.[19]

In Tarentum (southern Italy), Philolaos (480–? B.C.), was of the opinion that the heart carried the "generative force" (meaning emotions?), whereas the brain was the center of intelligence. In Croton (southern Italy), Alcmaeon (500–? B.C.), located all senses as well as the soul in the brain. He performed dissections, specifying the optic nerve and Eustachian tube in goats, as did Heracleitus (556–460 B.C.) in Ephesus (Asia Minor). No in-depth investigations followed, however, because it was considered bad fate for Greeks to be unburied and several city-states had severe punishments for those responsible for negligence in matters of the dead. Although dissections of criminals or abandoned children were not ruled out, anatomical or pathological study was not a routine practice.[20] The Greeks primarily observed the body from the outside, and Hippocrates (460–370 B.C.) made the most of the opportunity.

Lack of dissection resulted in an array of false statements. The Greeks found only twenty-two vertebrae instead of twenty-four; they thought the acromion was a separate bone; and they did not properly identify muscles. Tendons, vessels, and nerves were not distinguished (at least in the extremities). The parotid glands, the pancreas, and the lens of the eye were not even mentioned.[21] An author in the Hippocratic circle put the center of intellect in the left ventricle of the heart, from where the "rest of the soul" was to be governed, whereas another described the center of intellect, sensation, and motion in the brain.[22] Despite the conflicting views—which stemmed from lack of dissection and experiment—there is one basic difference between the Greeks and other ancient scientists: they always tried to explain things from what they saw—or thought they saw—without the interference of false premises.[23] In the Hippocratic writings, the following sentence gives the essence: "Divine is one as the other one. But everything happens according to Nature." Although common belief shrouded epilepsy in superstition—for instance, patients were warned against wearing black clothing or crossing their arms or legs, actions that were thought to foreshadow death—yet the followers of Hippocrates, meanwhile, argued: "Those who make epilepsy into a 'divine disease' [*morbus sacer*] are similar to present day magicians, sorcerers, charlatans and impostors who state that they are able to pull the moon from heavens, or extinguish the light of the sun, or create storm or sunshine, rain and draught."[24]

Noncommitted observation resulted in a number of superb descriptions and techniques as valid today as they were twenty-four hundred years ago: the Hippocratic face, premortem cyanosis, judging the temperature by the hand, employing percussion and ausculation, and descriptions of exanthemata, petechiae, jaundice, ascites, and the foamy sputum and sibilant rales of pulmonary edema. Hundreds of valuable signs were all witness to astute use of eyes, ears, palpation, and—last but not least—common sense. If we can forget for a second his lack of anatomical knowledge for sheer sober observation, we can go back to Hippocrates even today. What wonderful novelties would the ancient Greeks have brought to medicine had they some technological help and the opportunity to look into corpses stricken by disease.

The intellectual leaders in the fifth century B.C. gathered in Athens. Attention was withdrawn from the natural sciences and given to literature and ethics. The naturalists did not happen to reside in Athens: neither Democritus nor Hippocrates or their followers lived there. The eloquence of Socrates took over the scene, and his criticism of everything was persuasive. Siding with the aristocrats, he influenced the poor people regarding their inefficient or corrupt bureaucrats by saying: "It is absurd to choose magistrates by lot, where no one would dream of drawing lots for the pilot, a mason, a flute player, or any craftsman at all, though the shortcomings of such men are far less harmful, than those that disorder our government."[25] The logic of Socrates was convincing.

Xenophon, the historian, reflecting on his younger years, wrote, "Nothing was of greater benefit than to associate with Socrates and converse with him on any occasion, on any subject whatever," and in his later years, "In contemplating the man's wisdom and nobility of character, I find it beyond my power to forget him, or in remembering him to refrain from praising him."[26] Hippias, an opposing philosopher, countered him: "It is not enough that you laugh at others, questioning and refuting everybody, while you yourself are unwilling to give reason to anybody or to declare your opinion on any subject."[27]

Socrates approached things with the same uncommitted spirit as did Democritus or Hippocrates, going so far as to say: "Of the gods we know nothing." This view, of course, brought him to trial and death.[28] He studied human affairs and ethical questions at the expense of natural science, which he considered inscrutable. According to Will Durant: "Upon science his influence was injurious: Students were turned away from physical research and the doctrine of external design offered no encouragement to scientific analysis."[29]

Socrates had a great pupil-turned-promoter in Plato. His ethics and political thought, expounded with elegant style, made him the cherished philosopher of the Middle Ages and the Renaissance. His disciple and later rival Aristotle amassed a voluminous encyclopedia of knowledge touching all human activities. Nobody dared to criticize him for more than one thousand years, such was Aristotle's vast range of information. He was particularly interested in biology.

Aristotle sent his pupils to collect plants and animals, including information on their habits and breeding. On rare occurrences, he expressed interest in the appearance and conduct of people.[30] Alexander the Great, a former pupil, supplied him with species from the faraway lands of his military campaigns.[31] Aristotle was the first organizer and gatherer of the plant and animal world, and to show them to his students, he used diagrams and drawings in his lectures.

Aristotle's anatomy was based on animal dissections, and his physiology on speculative deductions and reiteration of old teachings. Although he performed a few experiments (with chicken embryos, for example, watching their development) and knew the color difference of blood in arteries and veins, he did not know anything about the physiology of respiration. He claimed that the liver and the spleen lacked any connection with the aorta; he did not distinguish nerves from tendons; and he attributed only eight pairs of ribs to humans. He thought that women had fewer teeth than men, and despite offering a fair description of the heart, he taught that the heart was the center of feeling and movements and that the only function of the brain was to excrete mucus.[32]

This was the state of the medical sciences in Athens toward the end of the fourth century B.C. as Plato's Academy and Aristotle's Lyceum set the pace in philosophy and the sciences.

Following the death of Alexander the Great in 323 B.C., however, rebellion arose against Macedonian rule. Aristotle, also a Macedonian and a favorite of Alexander's, was accused of impiety—with incalculable consequences. He thought it better to leave in order to avoid probable execution. Safe from persecution in a small Macedonian town in Thrace, he soon died in peace. For a long time the Mediterranean and the Near East suffered the ravages of bloody wars, broken treaties, and infamous leaders—except for a single city: Alexandria.

2

First Look into the Human Body, Third Century B.C.

AFTER THE DEATH of Alexander the Great in 323 B.C., his empire was divided into three areas by his most powerful generals. There were soon controversies over the inheritance: first, there were heated discussions; then, arguments and accusations; and, finally, open hostilities that lasted more than twenty years. At last in 307 B.C., Ptolemy I (called Soter the Savior) gained victory through diplomacy and a battle won by his friend Seleucus with four hundred elephants, trampling down the infantry of the enemy, reminiscent of tank battles in modern times.[1] The final settlement left Ptolemy with the most valuable shares of Alexander's heritage, Egypt and the cherished Aegean Islands, Cyprus and Rhodes, under his influence. He was declared king and god (descendent of Amon Rah), and coins were minted with his image on them, something not done in Egypt since the last pharaoh's death, two hundred years earlier.

Ptolemy Soter's education went back to the Macedonian king's court, where he was raised in close companionship with Alexander, and so he had been influenced by Aristotle. Gossip claimed that he was Alexander's half-brother, fathered by King Philip II, a notorious "ladies' man."[2] In later years Ptolemy wrote memoirs of his varied fortunes and misfortunes, regrettably lost in the turmoil of the times. With his background and literary inclinations, it was

11

natural that he would try to recruit scholars to his new capital, Alexandria. He invited Aristotle's successor, Theophrastus of Athens, but he declined. Meander, the famous writer of comedies, also refused the invitation, but not so Demetrius of Phaleron, statesman, orator, and governor who had been ousted from Athens. He gladly came to Alexandria as a refugee in 307 B.C. With his help and with the aid of the philosopher Strato, the Alexandrians set up a library and *mouseion,* a center honoring the muses, the goddesses of arts and sciences. The construction and beginning of the operation of that institution falls between the years 300 and 280 B.C.

The city of Alexandria had been founded by Alexander the Great in 332 B.C., approximately nine hundred years after the reign of Pharaoh Tutankhamen and two hundred years after the Persians invaded the country. Geographically, it was a well-chosen location at the westernmost branch of the Nile delta, protected by the almost uninhabited desert on the west. On the east the marshlands and numerous tributaries of the delta stretched for about fifty miles. The only way to approach the city would have been from the north by sea, or by taking a long detour toward the south through Memphis, near present-day Cairo, at the place where the Nile starts to break up to form the delta, approximately sixty miles from Alexandria. Outside forces did not have a good chance of attacking Alexandria.

Ptolemy was shrewd enough to secure the remains of Alexander the Great. He snatched the coffin from under the nose of his rivals with the pretext of supplying it with an "honor guard." By the time they realized that this was not his true motive, the remains of Alexander already had traveled toward Egypt, surrounded by strong military units. Alexander's body was put into a mausoleum in the center of the city, thus securing the mystique of his presence.

By the time the mouseion was established, a fairly large, thriving city already existed in place of the earlier fishing village. The mouseion and the library buildings were connected with beautiful marble colonnades, close to the royal palace with its surrounding parks, not far from the mausoleum of Alexander the Great. The mouseion itself had ten lecture halls, a botanical garden, and a zoo.[3] The two chief organizers, Demetrius and Strato, both favored the natural sciences.[4] Strato, follower of Anaxagoras and Epicurus, took over their fearless scrutiny of natural phenomena, which he tried to explain on the basis of natural causes rather than the actions of gods. Toward the end of the first Ptolemy's reign, a great scientific institution was ready with support of money and protection by the king in a wonderful setting in a beautiful city.

When Ptolemy Soter stepped down in 285 B.C. and gave place to his son, he handed over an empire that stretched from Egypt to the Greek islands. The ancient land of the pharaohs was rejuvenated by Greek enterprise, and the buzzing capital of Alexandria blended the old flavor with fresh spirit into a very heady mix. Meanwhile, Phoenicia and Rome were embroiled in a deadly struggle, and Persia became the province of friendly Seleucus. With its recently acquired provinces, Egypt was the only stable state in the Mediterranean-Mideast region.

The new king had lost his tutor Strato two years previously to Athens, where he had been invited to lead Aristotle's Lyceum. Demetrius, designer of the mouseion, was dismissed after Ptolemy II's ascent to the throne. The philosopher had committed a great mistake, for he favored the succession of the older son of Ptolemy I over the younger son, who became the king. Demetrius had to go, his previous achievements disregarded. Another surprise in court was more than an embarrassment: it was a shock. Ptolemy II had been married, but pressure from the Egyptian priests forced changes in his marital situation. The expected successor of a pharaoh had to show lineage to the god Amon Rah. But how could that be accomplished if there were an interruption of the pure blood of the king (deriving from the god) by an outsider, a queen not originated from Amon? There was only one solution: the king had to take a wife proven to be also a descendent of a god. Clear as a mathematical formula, the king had to marry his own sister. Ptolemy tried to avoid confrontation with the powerful priestly cast; consequently, he dismissed his first wife and married his sister, the previous queen of Macedon, acquiring from the scandalized Greeks the sarcastic name "Philadelphus," the "Sister Lover." By this act he showed that he honored the customs of Egypt and that he was worthy of support. He thus established the pattern followed by subsequent Ptolemies.

During his reign, Ptolemy Philadelphus had to defend his empire either by military means or shrewd diplomacy. All the temporary disturbances, however, affected only the periphery of his vast holdings. The capital Alexandria enjoyed peace, revenues from commerce, and a satisfactory administration.[5] In order to guide the traffic of the busy harbor, a lighthouse was built. The Pharos, four hundred feet high, its pillared cupola containing the flame most likely reflected by metal mirrors toward the ocean, showed the direction as far as thirty-eight miles.[6] It was cited as one of the Seven Wonders of the world. Ptolemy also had a canal dug between the Mediterranean and the Red Seas (precursor to the Suez Canal) that existed even to Roman times, thus opening commercial routes to India.[7] The waterways were protected by a navy consisting of thirty-five hundred warships, some of them quinqueremes (five rows of slaves pulling the oars), and the roads were patrolled by an army of 240,000 men.[8] Alexandria was made the safest seaport in the whole known world, and Egypt the wealthiest country.

Artists, musicians, and merchants flocked to Alexandria, coming from Greece proper, the Greek islands, the shores of Asia Minor, and southern Italy and Sicily.[9] Because all were Greeks, sharing the same language, they could join the discussion freely. On the meeting ground of so many origins, religions, and traditions, the ingrained "must" and "should" were weakened, and many points of views were discussed.

Ptolemy Philadelphus appointed Callimachus, an able poet and imaginative administrator, as chief librarian. Books were added to the original two hundred thousand scrolls collected largely by Demetrius, for the first time strictly cataloged alphabetically by authors; their biographical data and works were meticulously listed.[10] It was there that the works of Hippocrates were collected and classified.[11] Important foreign works were also translated, among them the Old Testament (referred to as the *Septuaginta* for the seventy-two Hebraic scholars who accomplished the task), in addition to Egyptian historical documents, Babylonian historical accounts, and astronomical and medical scripts.[12] The result was the melding of many cultures into one based on the Greek language, thus creating a new culture with a large and well-organized library without parallel.

The library was only one facet of the institution. The mouseion contained lecture halls, experimental buildings, dormitories where the scientists lived, and dining halls where they ate their meals while arguing, discussing, agreeing, or debating with each other. Prejudices were soon dropped voluntarily, or they were worn down. In the search for freedom of thought and study, but also for a better life, people came from all corners of the world. The scientists received their salaries from the king's treasury because he himself was interested in promoting knowledge in the natural sciences.

With the interest in biology and mathematics, as well as Babylonian astronomical knowledge, Alexandrian science became fact-oriented. The influence of Socrates and Plato, who were disinterested in the material world, faded to make way for inquiry into matter, or the universe by observation and measurement. A heliocentric hypothesis was soon postulated by Aristarchus, who also estimated the distance of the moon from the earth, albeit incorrectly, and the size of the moon almost correctly.[13] Similar views almost ended the life of Anaxagoras in Athens 170 years earlier, for he was accused of impiety and atheism. The achievements of Euclid in geometry and Archimedes in mathematics, as well as the invention of mechanical optical devices, were made in those decades in Alexandria.

In medicine the same approach prevailed. For the first time in history, the study of human anatomy was practiced systematically. Previously, opening the human body was deemed sacrilegious by all cultures, except in Egypt where mummification was a religious ceremony rather than a scientific practice. The Egyptian priests who put the viscera into containers did not search structures for knowledge; they performed their rituals according to their religious texts dealing with the afterlife. In contrast, the Greek scientists' goal was to satisfy their curiosity about the workings of human organs.

Celsus, a Roman author of medical works some centuries later (first century A.D.), wrote: "Herophilus and Erasistratus . . . laid open men while still alive, criminals received out of the prisons from the king, and while these were still breathing, they observed parts which beforehand nature had concealed, their position, color, shape, size, arrangement, hardness, substance, smoothness, relation, process and depressions of each and whether any part is inserted or received by an other one."[14] We shudder at this report.

To make convicted criminals available for study—they were to be executed anyway—might not have been regarded as harsh for a culture that was used to seeing the killing of rivals by the highest ranks of society, let alone the routine application of the death penalty and torture.[15] Celsus must have obtained his information from the followers of the Alexandrian anatomists whose teachings had quite a number of supporters in Rome. Widespread medical groups listened to their masters' opinions even centuries later, and it is not likely that they distorted facts about the founders of their doctrines.

Herophilus started his dissections of humans, including fetuses, in the time of Ptolemy Soter around 290 B.C. He correctly described the liver and compared its shape in different animal species. He gave the name *duodenum* and described the chyle vessels eighteen hundred years before they were rediscovered by Aselli.[16] He also described the ovaries, the uterus, and the cervix correctly. He demonstrated the Fallopian tube and gave sound opinions in obstetrics. His greatest discoveries were made in the nervous system. The brain was finally given its proper place as the organ of sensation and command (although he thought the center was the fourth ventricle), contrary to the teachings of his professor Praxagoras and Aristotle himself, who thought these functions were related to the heart. He demonstrated that the nerves originated from the brain and spinal cord and that they are not the small vessels his teacher thought them to be but instead transmitters of voluntary motion to the muscles. This new notion, at long last, straightened out the confusion that mixed nerves with arteries and tendons. Most likely by cutting and touching nerves, he identified sensory as well as motor nerves.[17] He was the first to specify the three membranes covering the brain, and he also distinguished the cerebrum from the cerebellum. He established the confluence of the sinuses (*torcular Herophili*), the choroid plexuses, the ventricles and the *calamus scriptorius,* the eye with the choroid, the vitreous, and the retina— quite a chain of discoveries, all because he was the first to open the skull and examine it.

Herophilus correctly emphasized the great difference between the walls of the arteries and the veins, pointed out the connection between heartbeat and pulse, counted the pulse rate exactly with the recently developed clock (clepsydra), and distinguished the heart's strength, size, and rhythm.[18] He called the pulmonary artery the "artery-like vein" and the pulmonary veins the "vein-like arteries," either because of their relationship to adjacent vessels on the right and on the left or because of the color of the blood they contained, similar to the "real" arteries and veins. None of his writings have survived, unfortunately; his work is known only through brief references and short commentaries by other writers.

Erasistratus, a somewhat younger contemporary of Herophilus, had a distinguished connection to Aristotle. Some claim he married Aristotle's daughter.[19] He ended up in the court of Seleucus, being a friend of his son Antiochus, and spent a number of years in Antiochia, the capital city of the Seleucid empire (present-day Antachia, Syria). It was not a quiet place. Year by year war, invasion by hostile armies, family feuds, assassinations, and revolts followed each other in fast sequence. Alexandria, in contrast, offered security instead of turmoil and uncertainty; only there could Erasistratus have had the opportunity to perform human dissections.[20] There was no other place to pursue such ends.

According to Galen, only in his later years did Erasistratus end up in Alexandria in the Ptolemaic court.[21] Erasistratus expanded on the work of Herophilus. Comparing the brain in different animal species and humans, he observed: "Just as deer, hare and any other animal that greatly excels the others in running, is well provided with muscles, tendons and nerves, so man since he is superior to all other animals in intelligence, has a very convoluted brain."[22]

His description of the chordae tendineae in the cardiac ventricles and his declaration that the heart, not the liver, is the center of the arteries and veins were correct.[23] The supposition of connections between veins and arteries (*synanastomoses*), a vague guess of the capillaries (although they functioned, according to him, only in disease), was a novel concept. Up until his time, the veins were supposed to carry blood and the arteries *pneuma* (air?) in centrifugal direction to the organs and not communicate with each other.[24] The cardiac valves were described in detail, and he noted: "They turn from the inside outwards so as to open the mouths of the vessels [aorta and pulmonary artery] under pressure of the matter flowing out on the occasion when the heart distributes matter. But for all the time they firmly close the mouths of the vessels and do not permit any of the expelled matter to return."

Being a mechanically minded scientist, Erasistratus described the heart as a pump that "expanding like a smith's bellows draws matter in, through its extension (diastole)."[25] With such clear-cut knowledge of heart contraction and valve function, he explained the moving of "matter" in correct pressure-related mechanics; his error was that he thought *pneuma,* not blood, was present in the left ventricle. And on the right? Flow of blood from the liver to the periphery was contrary to this logic, but ingrained teachings of the time influenced his explanations. Again his personal views can be traced back only through references and not his own description. Even so, we know by his astute observation that he recognized that the expansion of the arteries coincides with the contraction of the heart, contrary to the earlier belief that the expansion of the arteries and the heart are simultaneous.[26] Detailed description of the aorta, the gastric arteries, the vena cava and hepatic veins, the azygos vein, the portal vein, and the premonition of the vasa vasorum were all discoveries of the greatest merit.[27]

Dissections and vivisections led Erasistratus to observe the function of the epiglottis, the gastric peristalsis. True to himself, he did not fall victim to the authority of Hippocrates with his four humors, but recognized only the two he could see, namely, the blood and the bile. He took advantage of the knowledge he accumulated with his anatomical studies: he operated on inguinal hernia and cataract, and extracted calculi from the urinary bladder.[28] He put a curve in straight catheters, initiating the S-shaped "male catheter"—used until it was replaced with the flexible rubber catheter two thousand years later. He may have conducted post-mortems to study the place from which a disease took its toll: he observed the liver to be hard in cases of ascites and concluded that there must be a constant relationship of this kind. He believed that organs, not humors, were the origin of diseases. He "cut into the skin and membrane over the liver and applied drugs to surround the organ completely, then while boldly lying bare the affected part, he purged the bowel"—a crude version of our organ-oriented efforts.[29]

When Ptolemy Philadelphus died in 247 B.C., a storm broke loose. The tranquility of more than thirty years of Alexandrian life was interrupted. The third Ptolemy warred against Syria.[30] The conflict continued for years and took him to the shores of Asia Minor, the Aegean Islands, Thrace, and Persia, far away from Egypt. Meanwhile, an unpleasant situation arose in the homeland: the yearly inundation of the Nile failed to occur, resulting in food shortages. Riots broke out, fueled by the priests' complaints about the long absence of the king: the first civil disturbance in Alexandria. The king returned and resolved that he never again would leave the country. Hostile sentiments were calmed down.[31] Still, whether it was sheer coincidence or the uncertainties of existence, it was in those years that Archimedes accepted an invitation to Syracuse (Sicily) and Erasistratus also left the city and died on the island of Samos.

Ptolemy III supported the library and selected the distinguished astronomer Eratosthenes to become chief librarian. Among other things, he was famous for calculating the size of the equator (missing by only fifty miles) and making a map of 675 stars, using only the naked eye.[32] Under the leadership of Eratosthenes the Alexandrian library far surpassed any other library in the known world. It represented the largest collection of books anywhere with seven hundred thousand items. Ptolemy III was "so jealous for the reputation of his library" that he issued an order that all books found on ships unloading in the harbor were to be seized and only copies returned to the owners.[33] The originals thus acquired received a special label "from the ship." The king's collection mania resulted in forgeries arriving from the book markets of Athens and Rhodes to milk the royal treasury.

Discoveries in anatomy furthered medicine considerably. Ligation of bleeding vessels began to be practiced, instead of burning the bleeders. Anesthesia was achieved with mandrake, a plant that contains scopolamine and hyoscyamine. Its use caused amnesia for the unpleasant memories of an operation. The discoverers and the dates of these innovations are not known to us, but they originated in Alexandria in the second half of the third century B.C.[34] At the same time a follower of Herophilus named Mantias and his younger associate Heracleides of Tarentum (Sicily), who later became famous, performed experiments with drugs, and the symptoms of opium consumption were well known to them. On the basis of these experiments Heracleides wrote extensively on poisons and medicaments and about their preparation and study. The achievements of the natural scientists in Alexandria were more factual and substantial than those of the famous earlier scholars of Athens.

We started to wake up to reality about the Universe and about our body and its functions. It was a triumph of reason, the first short-lived triumph.

Musculoskeletal Images

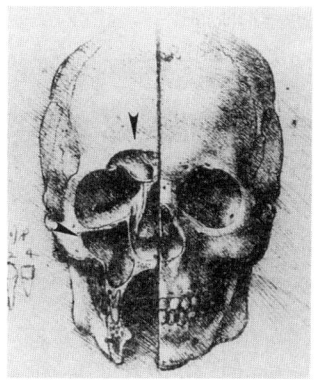

1. First depiction of paranasal sinuses, by Leonardo da Vinci, 1489. From Leonardo da Vinci, *I manoscritti di Leonardo da Vinci della Reale Biblioteca di Windsor: Dell'anatomia Fogli B,* trans. G. Piumati (Turin: Roux and Viarengo, 1901), 41v.

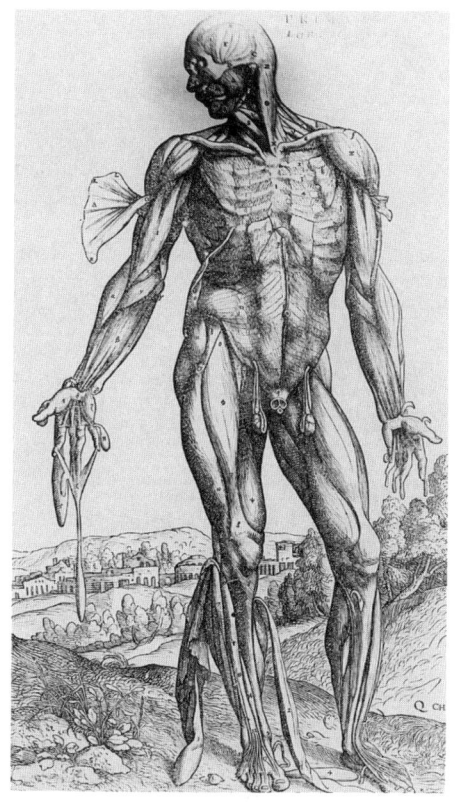

2. Muscle man of Vesalius, 1543. From Andreas Vesalius, *De Humani Corporis Fabrica Libri Septem* (Basil: Ex Officina Ioannis Oporini, 1543).

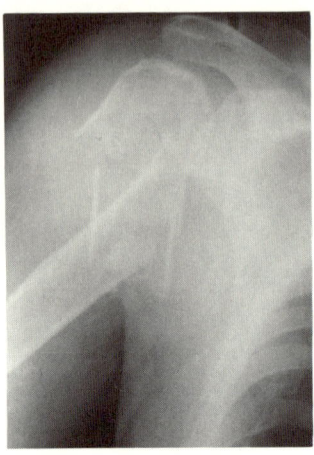

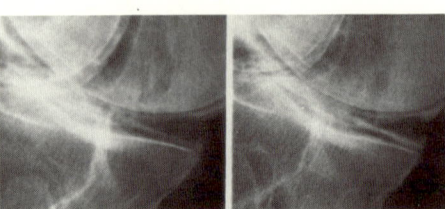

4. Knee arthrogram with water-soluble contrast material, as practiced since the 1950s.

3. X-ray picture of shoulder on glass plate, 1910. Note the poor contrast and lack of muscle definition.

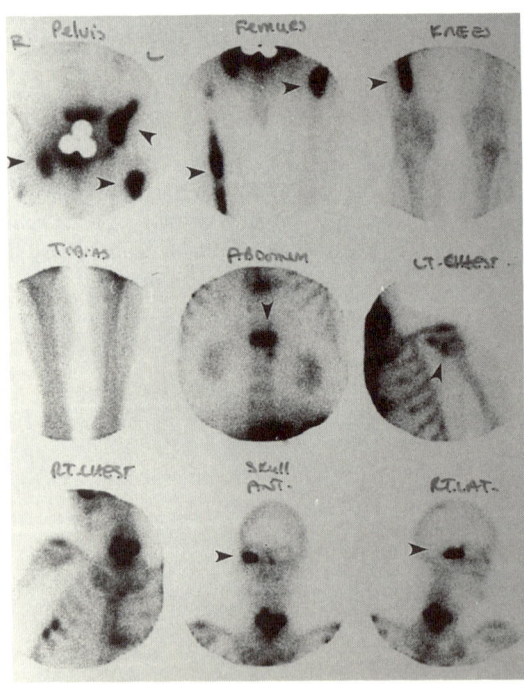

5. Bone scan with Anger camera showing metastases, post-1958.

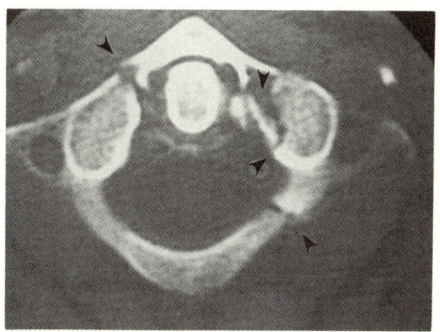

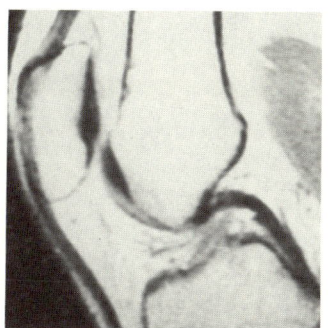

6. CT image of spine with fractures, post-1973.

7. MR image of knee, with tendons, cartilage, and muscles well visualized, mid-1980s.

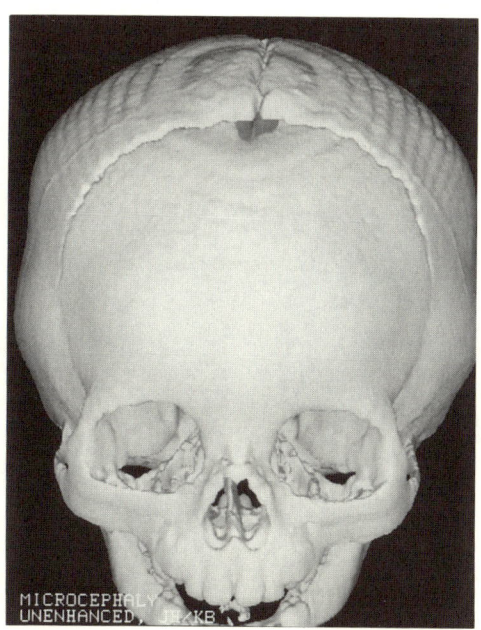

8. Microcephaly with three-dimensional CT technique, 1995. From J. H. Scatliff, M.D., University of North Carolina, Chapel Hill.

Cardiovascular Images

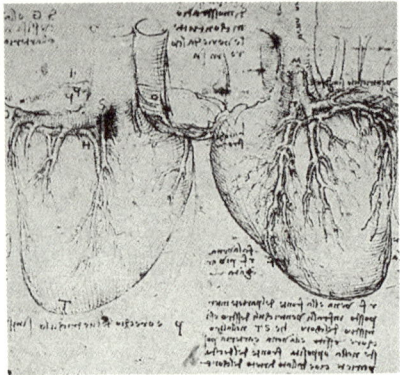

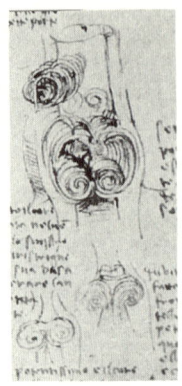

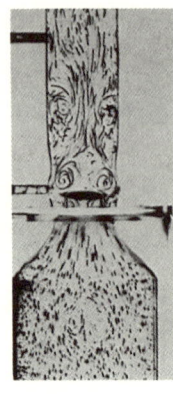

9. Sketches of the heart by Leonardo da Vinci, 1513. From Leonardo da Vinci, *Quaderni d'Anatomia,* ed. and trans. O. C. L. Vangensten, A. Fonahn, and H. Hopstock (Christiania: J. Dybwad, 1911–1916), 2:4r.

10. *Left,* simulated hemodynamics in glass model of aorta by Leonardo da Vinci, 1513. From Leonardo da Vinci, *Quaderni d'Anatomia,* 2:13v.

11. *Right,* simulated hemodynamics in glass model by Wieting, 1972. From H. Greenfield and W. Kolff, "The Prosthetic Heart Valve and Computer Graphics," *JAMA* 219 (1972): 69–74. © 1972, American Medical Association.

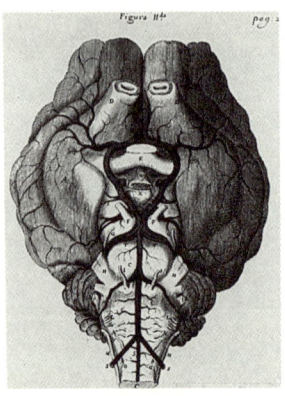

12. Circle of Willis, based on color injection in sheep, drafted by Christopher Wren, 1664. From Thomas Willis, *Cerebri Anatome: Cui Accessit Nervorum Descriptio et Usus Studio Thoma Willis* (London: J. Martyn and J. Allestry, 1664).

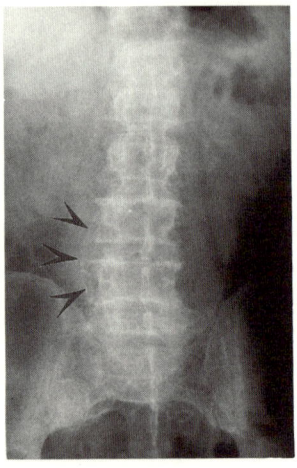

13. Aortic aneurysm; calcifications in the wall could be seen only after the 1910s.

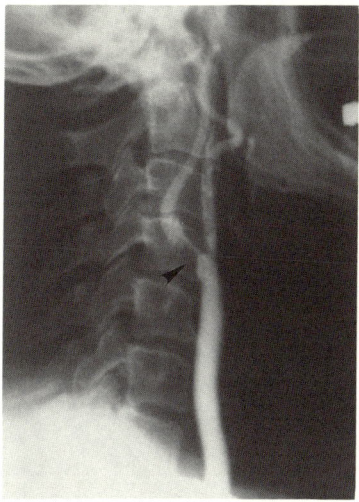

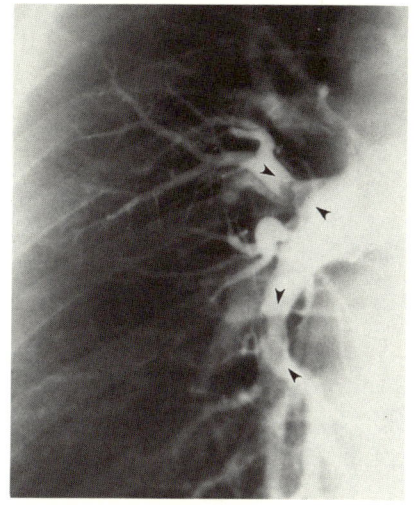

14. Angiogram of atheromatous
plaque in internal carotid, post-1930.

15. Pulmonary angiogram showing
several emboli, post-1930.

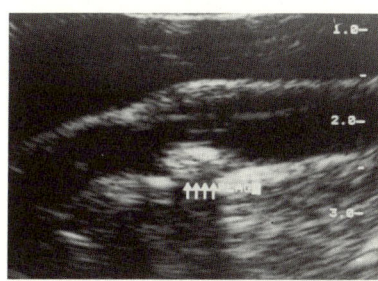

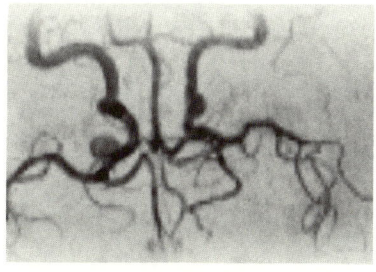

16. Ultrasound image of atheromatous
plaque in internal carotid, 1970s.

17. MRI angiogram of aneurysm of the
posterior communicating artery, 1995.
From J. H. Scatliff, M.D., University
of North Carolina, Chapel Hill.

Respiratory System Images

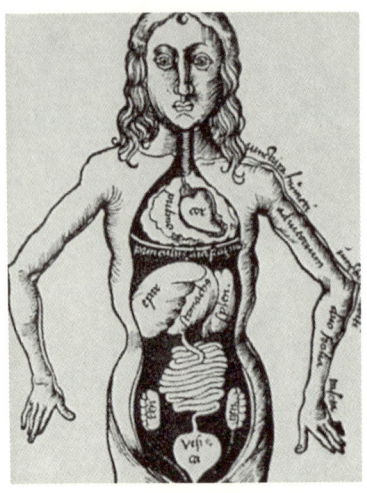

18. "Margarita Philosophica," from a 1504 encyclopedia. From Gregor Reisch, *Margarita Philosophica* (Freiburg: Joannia Schotti Argentinen, 1504).

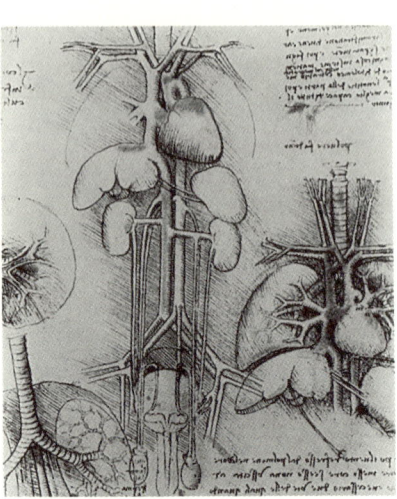

19. Thoracic and abdominal vessels, showing an inaccurate connection of pulmonary veins with vena cava, by Leonardo da Vinci, 1507. From Leonardo da Vinci, *Quaderni d'Anatomia,* ed. and trans. O. C. L. Vangensten, A. Fonahn, and H. Hopstock (Christiania: J. Dybwad, 1911–16), 3:10v.

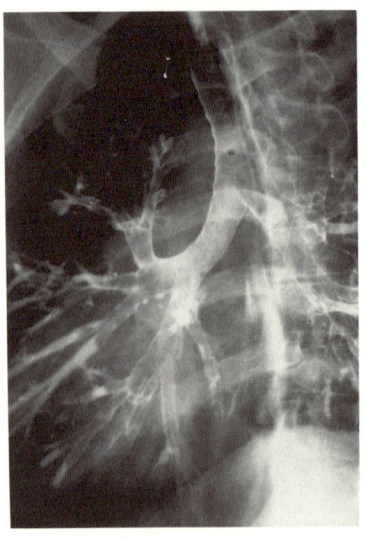

20. Bronchogram, post-1920s.

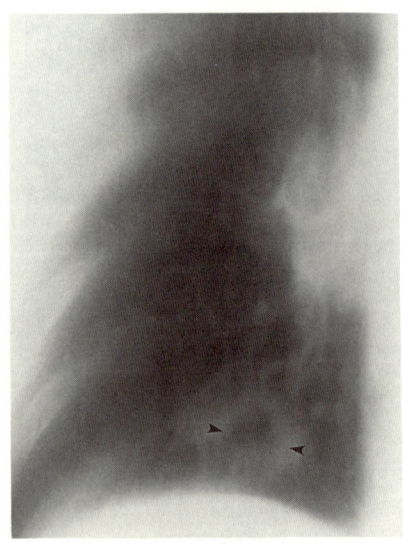

21. Conventional tomography showing abscess cavity in lung, early 1940s.

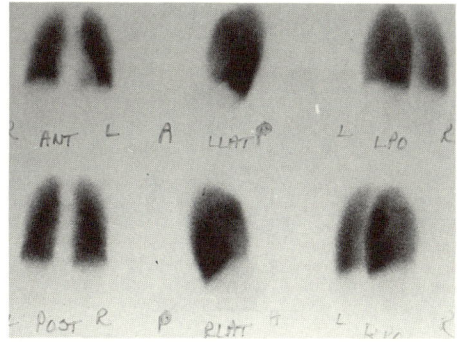

22. Perfusion nuclear study of the lung, post-1960s.

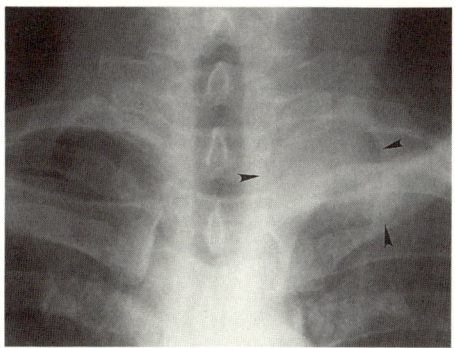

23. Superior sulcus tumor with film-screen technique, the standard approach, 1920s.

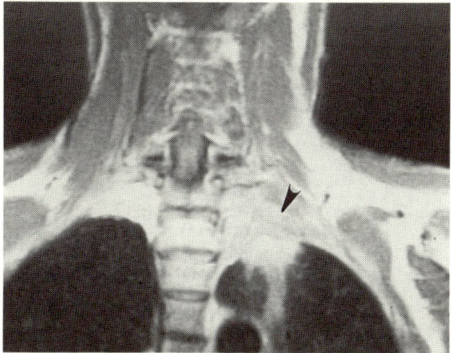

24. Superior sulcus tumor by MR image, mid-1980s. Note clear definition of details compared to the film-screen image.

Gastrointestinal Images

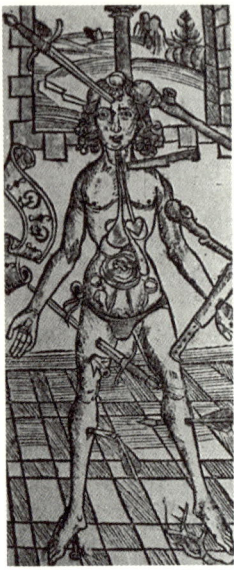

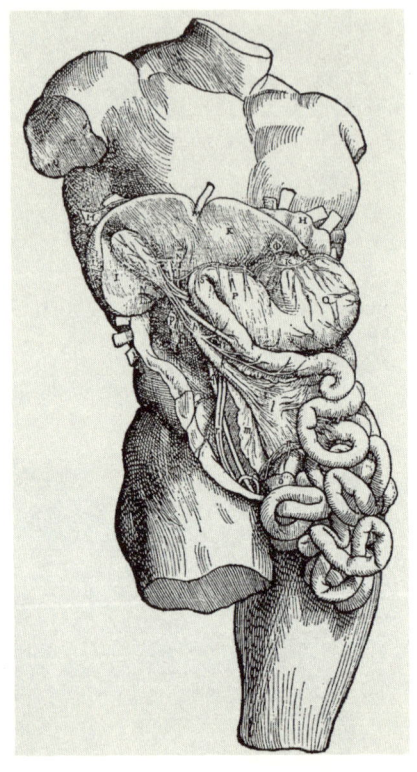

25. Medical illustration from Hieronymus Brunschwig, *Dis ist das Buch der Cirurgia: Hantwirckung der Wundartzny vo Hyeroimo Brauschwig, Buch der Chirurgia* (Augsburg: J. Schonsperger, 1497).

26. Stomach, small bowels, liver, and gall bladder in book of Vesalius, 1543. From Andreas Vesalius, *De Humani Corporis Fabrica Libri Septem* (Basil: Ex Officina Ioannis Oporini, 1543).

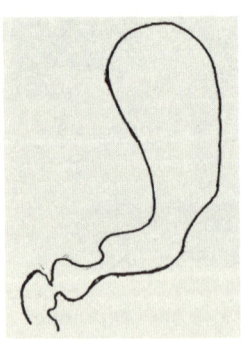

27. Line drawing of stomach, taken post-1910 fluoroscopy screen. Contemporary long exposures would have blurred outlines badly.

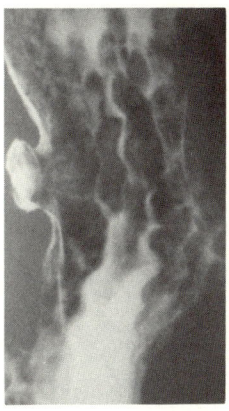

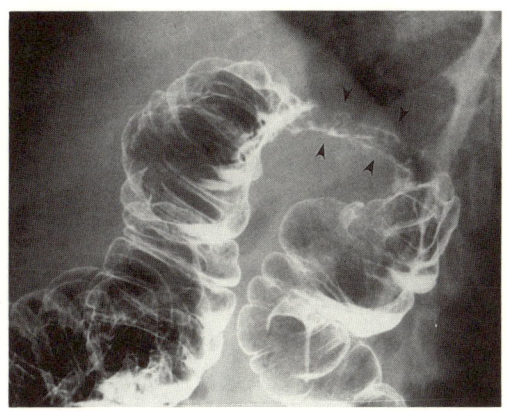

28. Gastric ulcer with nice mucosal folds, taken with "new" Coolidge tube, post-1920s.

29. Double-contrast enema image of narrowing of the colon due to carcinoma, post-1920s.

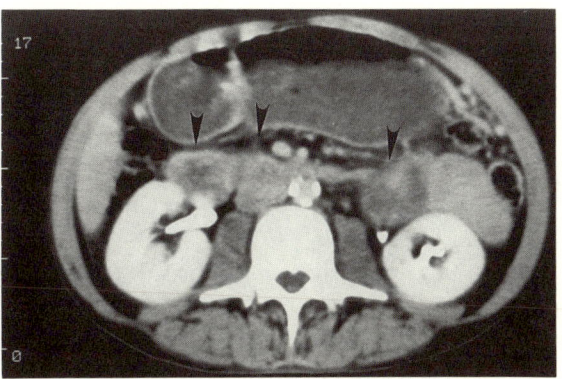

30. CT scan of enlarged malignant retroperitoneal lymph nodes, late 1970s.

Genitourinary Tract Images

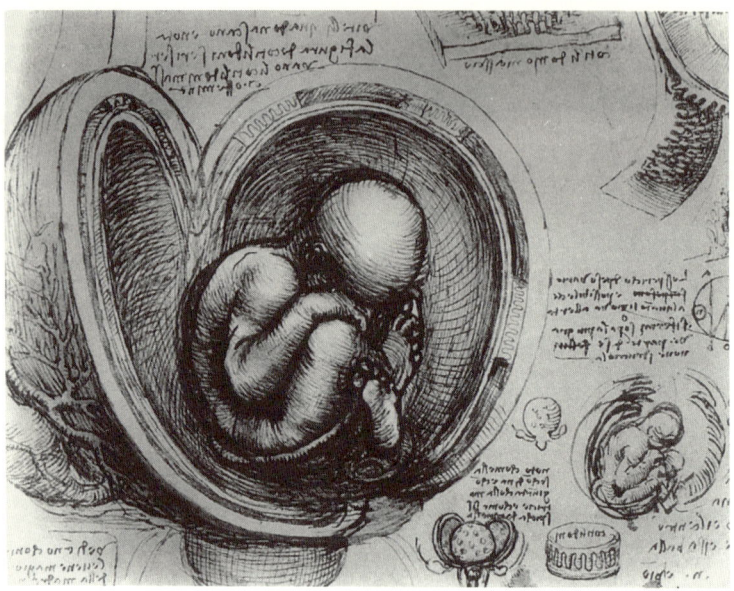

31. Fetus in utero, by Leonardo da Vinci, 1512. From Leonardo da Vinci, *Quaderni d'Anatomia,* ed. and trans. O. C. L. Vangensten, A. Fonahn, and H. Hopstock (Christiania: J. Dybwad, 1911–16), 3:8r.

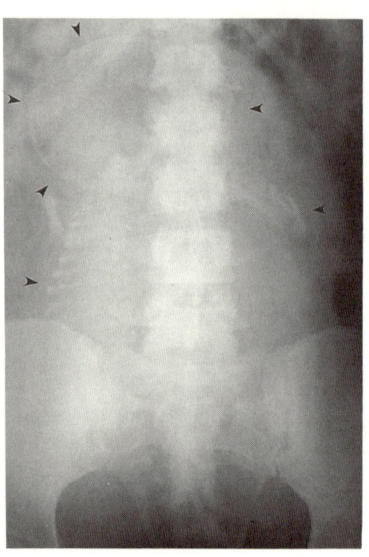

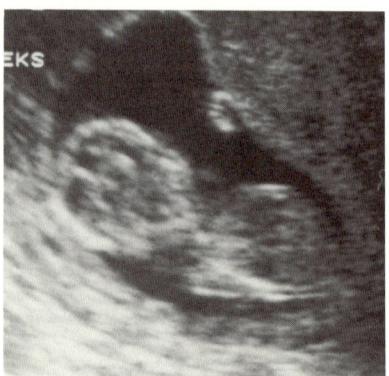

33. Ultrasound image of fetus with umbilical cord in uterine cavity, late 1970s.

32. Fetus in plain abdominal film, showing poor definition of fetal bones, post-1910.

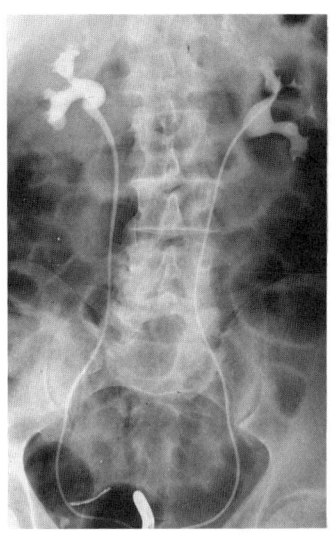

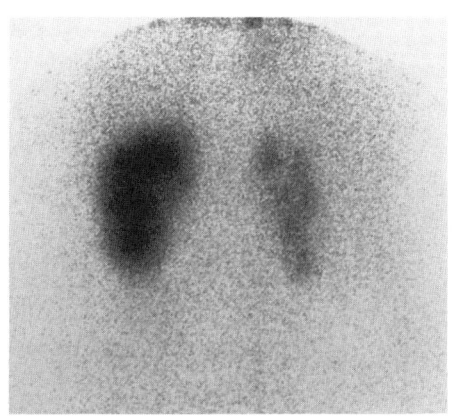

35. Nuclear study depicting shrinking of left kidney due to chronic infection, post-late-1950s.

34. Retrograde pyelogram, with various contrast materials, post-1910s.

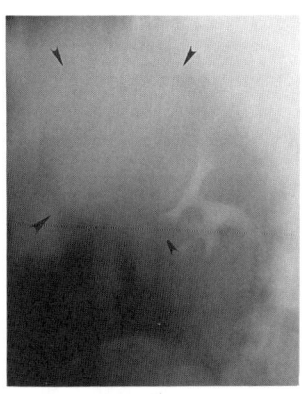

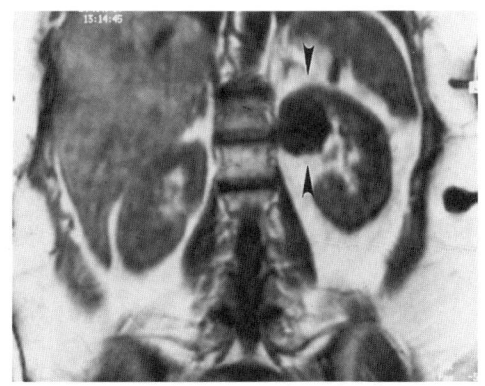

36. Conventional tomogram of kidney, in which cyst or tumor cannot be distinguished, post-1930.

37. MR image of kidney tumor, mid-1980s.

Organ Images

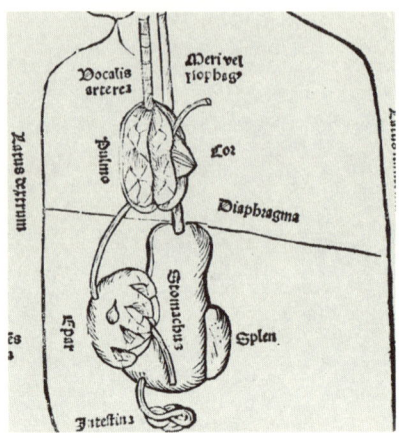

38. Abdominal organs depicted in 1499. From Johannes Peyligk, *Compendium Philosophiae Naturalis* (Leipzig: Melchior Lotter, 1499).

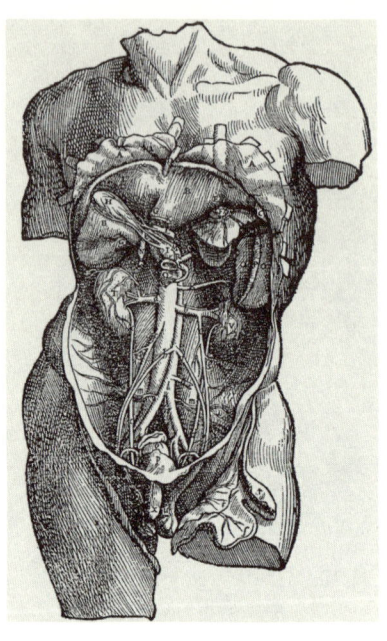

39. Abdominal organs in book of Vesalius, 1543. From Andreas Vesalius, *De Humani Corporis Fabrica Libri Septem* (Basil: Ex Officina Ioannis Oporini, 1543).

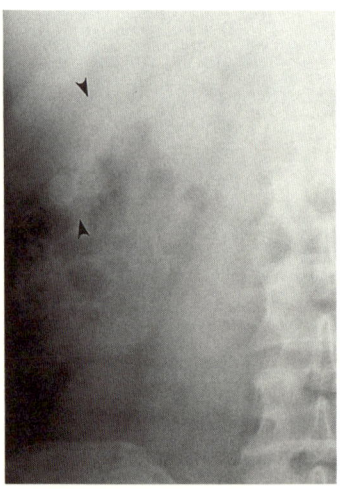

40. Only calcified gall stones could be shown before 1920s.

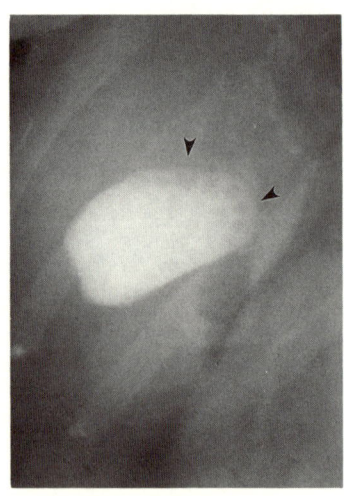

41. Gall stones without calcifications, as shown with the Graham-Cole test, post-1923.

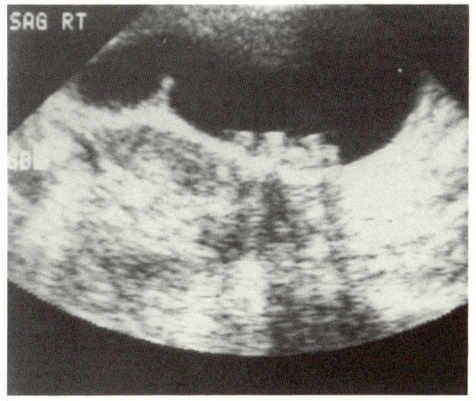

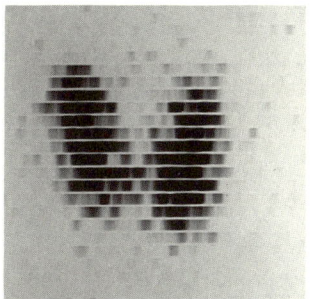

43. Rectilinear thyroid scan, 1950s.

42. Ultrasound image of gall stones, post-1970s.

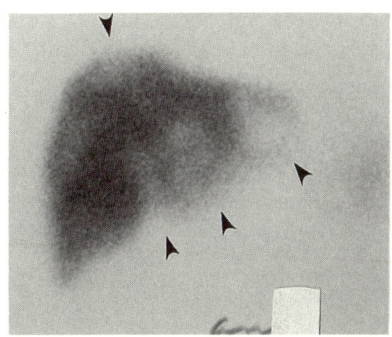

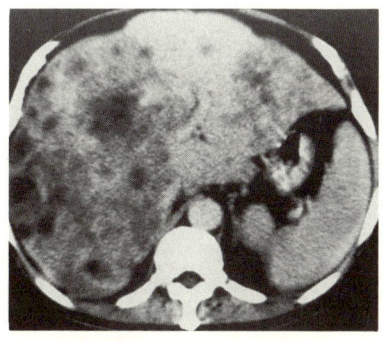

44. Nuclear study of liver metastases, 1960s.

45. CT scan of liver metastases, mid-1970s.

Nervous System Images

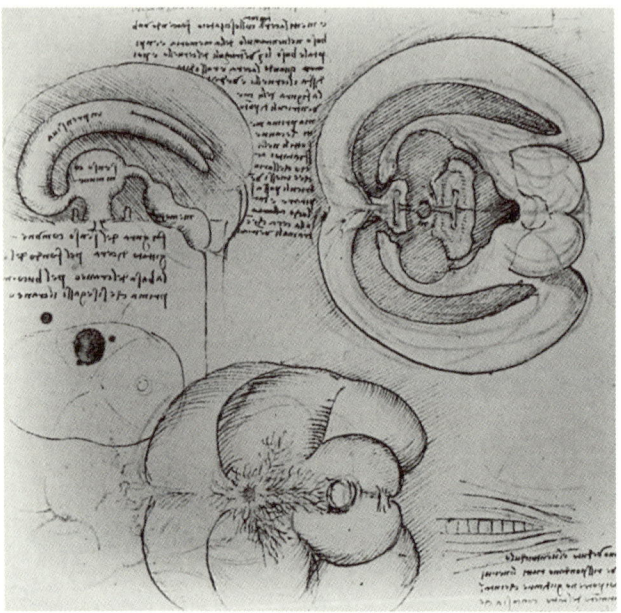

46. Wax cast of cerebral ventricles in ox by Leonardo da Vinci, 1507. From Leonardo da Vinci, *Quaderni d'Anatomia,* ed. and trans. O. C. L. Vangensten, A. Fonahn, and H. Hopstock (Christiania: J. Dybwad, 1911–16), 5:7r.

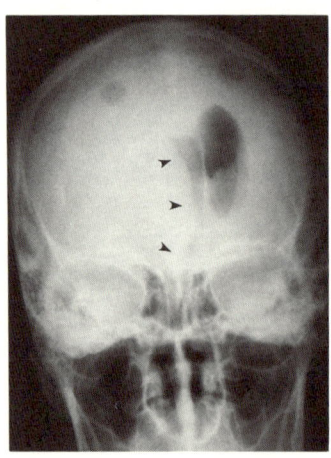

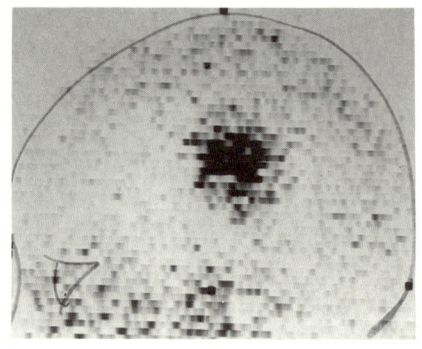

48. Linear scan of brain tumor, from a nuclear study, 1960s.

47. Dandy's ventriculogram technique, showing displacement of midline structures by tumor, post-1916.

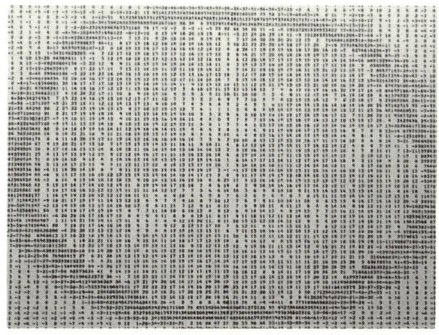

49. CT image of brain, showing absorption coefficients by numbers, 1973. From J. Ambrose and G. Hounsfield, "Computerized Transverse Axial Tomography," *British Journal of Radiology* 46 (1973): 148–49.

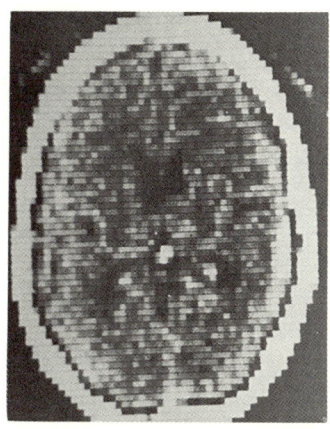

50. CT scan of brain with early equipment, 1973. From J. Ambrose and G. Hounsfield, "Computerized Transverse Axial Tomography," *British Journal of Radiology* 46 (1973): 148–49.

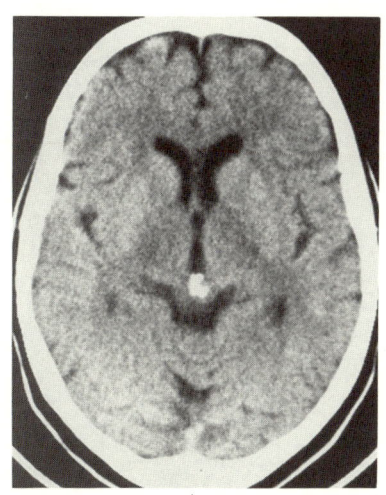

51. CT scan of brain with more advanced equipment, 1980s.

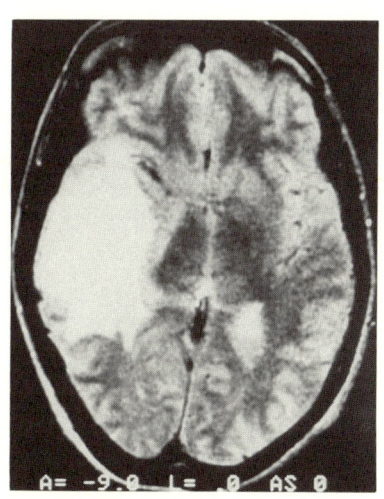

52. MR image of large temporal infarct, mid-1980s.

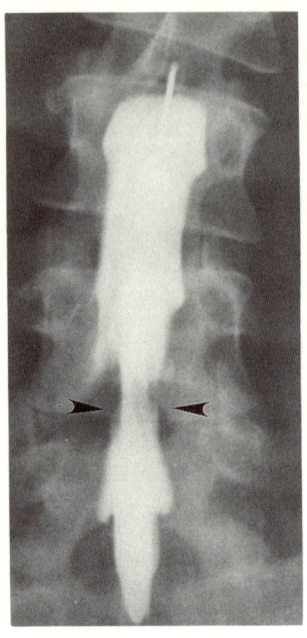

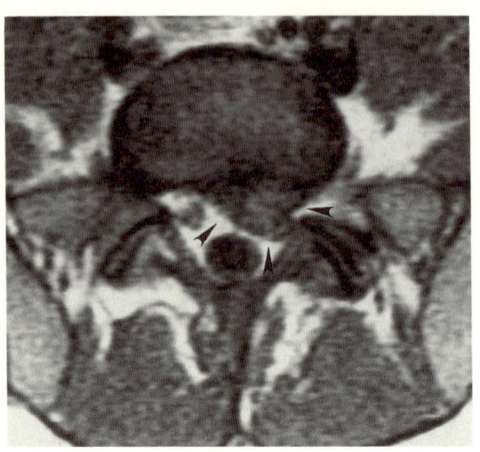

54. MR image of herniated disc, 1980s.

53. Myelogram of herniated
disk, post-1923.

3

Years of Stagnation, 200 B.C.–A.D. 1450

WHEN KING PTOLEMY III died in 221 B.C., the golden days of Alexandria came to an end. Ptolemy IV came under the influence of an evil Greek advisor, Agathocles, whose sister established herself as the royal mistress. Their intrigues resulted in the murders of Ptolemy IV's brother, uncle, and even his mother, all allegedly with his knowledge.[1] The monarch also began drinking heavily. In the midst of that internal disarray, war began between Egypt and Syria. In Raphia, a few miles south of present-day Gaza, Ptolemy IV won a decisive victory in 217 B.C. with the help of native troops. Up to that time only Macedonians and Greeks had fought for the Ptolemies. Egyptian participation in the victory naturally had the immediate result of demand for land, better official positions, and court favors for native persons. Tensions between Egyptians and the Greek-Macedonian element in the Nile Delta erupted in revolt. When Ptolemy IV died in 203 B.C., the civil war was still going on.

The heir, Ptolemy V, was only five years old. Agathocles and his sister saw the opportunity to take over. The only obstacle to their scheme was the popular queen mother whom they eliminated by murder. But when the people found out about the plot, they demanded that Agathocles and his family be handed over. "All being delivered together into the hands of the mob," according to Polybius, the historian, "some began to bite them, some to stab them, others to gouge out their eyes. They tore each body as it fell limb from limb, until they mutilated them all. For the inhabitants of Egypt are capable of terrible violence."[2]

Life for the scientists in the mouseion must have become unstable and fraught with doubts about the future. Their findings and their way of thinking were discredited. Adverse views began to circulate: Dissections are unimportant. For what end are they helpful? Interest should not be directed to that which produces illness but to that which cures it.[3] Such attitudes challenged the "Let us see first" mentality, allowing the culture to slip back to old practices. Superstition and quackery returned to dominate Egypt. Soon crocodile feces as a remedy became popular again, so much so that imitations were sold in the black market.[4]

At the same time, Greek supremacy was slipping. Egyptian natives were appointed to offices that in previous generations were only open to Greeks.[5] Meanwhile, prices were rising and overseas migration from Greek cities became increasingly difficult. Uncertainty prevailed in the Mediterranean on account of the Second Punic War of 218–201 B.C. At its end, Hannibal was driven back by the Romans, Spain became a Roman province, and the whole Mediterranean came more and more under Roman influence. In addition to internal difficulties—or probably as a consequence of them—Egypt in 198 B.C. lost Syria and the Aegean Islands the following year. The decline of commerce and the loss of tax revenue had a dramatic effect.[6] The usual silver coins were replaced by copper, and a number of high offices were sold to Syrians and Egyptians to generate income.[7] Alexandria became a different city.

The atmosphere of the mouseion deteriorated. To be a scholar in Alexandria became less attractive, possibly even dangerous. Only as an aging witness to better days, the illustrious astronomer, Eratosthenes, lived through twenty-five more troubled years. The circumstances of his death are not to be neglected: blind and doubtless depressed by the changes in the mouseion, he committed suicide in 197 B.C. The struggle between the king and his brother led to a situation in which nobody really knew whom to follow. The administration that was once so sound and so envied by all the ancient world lost honor.[8]

The creative years of Alexandria had passed. They lasted just about fifty years (295–246 B.C.), with such scientists as Strato, the natural philosopher, mathematicians Euclides and Archimedes, Aristarchus, proponent of the solar system, and Herophilus and Erasistratus, the medical investigators. A rare assembly of talent, all had enjoyed a favorable peaceful environment and supportive rulers. In the twilight of that glory another fifty years were experienced in a less calm but still tolerable atmosphere, with astronomer Eratosthenes and pharmacologic experimenter Heracleides. Later, as circumstances deteriorated, no further achievements can be pinpointed. Only the library remained as the frozen transmitter of past activities.

Toward the middle of the second century B.C. the remaining Greeks in Alexandria were of "mixed breed." As Polybius states: "They have largely disappeared chiefly owing to Ptolemy Fiscon [the "Fat One," Ptolemy VII], who, when revolted against, let loose his troops over and over again on the population and massacred them."[9] Teachers in the mouseion were intimidated or chased out of the city. In 145 B.C. the chief librarian actually fled for his life. One of the "spear men"—another word for army officers—was appointed to the vacant post that had once been held by the most brilliant scholars.[10]

After the Romans took over in 46 B.C., the confusion of the late Ptolemies gave way to a more orderly management, although the original zeal of the mouseion scholars was no longer to be found. Yet leading physicians of those days (first and second century B.C. and first century A.D.) living in Rome or in cities of the Greek "colonies" were still trained in Alexandria, which had the best scientific library in the world. However, most of the library holdings consisted of the commentaries of Hippocrates or other past great medical researchers rather than contemporary writings. Many times these physicians' energies were expended through polemics, not findings, as they fought over passages of books. The eminent physician of the first century A.D., Rufus of Ephesus, deplored the absence of human dissections.[11] The only surviving aspect of the study of human anatomy was a single skeleton shown to physicians who still flocked to Alexandria, because to acquire position or fame in medicine one had to spend time there, no matter how overbearing and dogmatic the teachers had become, as the young physician from Pergamon (present-day Bergama, Turkey), Galen, described them to be.[12]

After having spent some years in Alexandria, Galen returned to his native city on the shore of Asia Minor, only to try his luck a little later in Rome, in A.D. 161. Soon he became known to the important leaders. He held public demonstrations of animal dissections and other experiments. He became embroiled in bitter debates frequently, partly because of his superior knowledge and partly because of his nature—it almost seemed as though he welcomed challenge for the opportunity to abuse others. When a great epidemic of plague accompanied returning troops in A.D. 166, not waiting their arrival in Rome, he quickly returned to Pergamon. His fame, however, was established in Rome, and the new emperor, Marc Aurel, summoned him back. Reluctantly, Galen returned to Rome when the plague was past. He became personal physician to the son of the emperor, Commodus, who succeeded his father, and later to the next ruler, Septimius Severus. When Galen died in A.D. 200, he was the uncontested authority in medicine.

Both theory and practice, as he knew it, were put down in his encyclopedic compilation of four hundred books of which eighty-three are extant. Although he gave his opinions on dietetics, the doctrines of Hippocrates and Plato, the composition of medicines according to locality, and the nature of man, we will concentrate only on his contributions to the visible in medicine. He did not have an opportunity to dissect human corpses, and he was not interested in surgery. In fact, he had a "deep distaste" for it.[13] On the other hand, through his experiments and animal dissections, he made great steps forward in physiology (the use of parts, as he expressed it) and in anatomy.

In animals Galen described the main landmarks of the brain, as already known to Alexandrians, but added the corpora quadrigemina, hypophysis, infundibulum, the vermiform process. He noted not only seven pairs of cerebral nerves (of the twelve we know) but added the sympathetic ganglia as "reinforcers of the nerves."[14] He transected the spinal cord all across or halfway, causing paraplegia or hemiplegia, and produced aphonia by cutting the recurrent nerve.[15] When the fifth cervical nerve was cut, he observed paralysis of the subscapular muscle, the scalenus, and the pectoralis muscles. This seems rather uninteresting, but at a time when experiments were not performed (except by the Alexandrians), Galen's approach was unique. His working practice was to cause a lesion, to interrupt something in the body, and then watch what happened and relate that to clinical experience or to symptoms he saw at the bedside. That method had never been used before. He was going against ingrained concepts, against the stone wall of general acceptance. For instance, some of the ancients held that the nerves derived from the heart. Galen found that when he cut the cervical nerves, the heart stopped beating. This meant that the impulse of movement came from the spine toward the heart, not from the heart to the spine. With this simple experiment he overthrew centuries, nay, thousands of years, of false belief.[16]

His other contributions in experimental physiology were made in the cardiovascular system. He observed that the heart showed movements after it had been cut out of its place—in other words, without nervous supply—showing some kind of independence. Furthermore, he proved that arteries contain blood, contrary to the teaching of Erasistratus, who thought they contained pneuma (air). He was certainly not the only scientist to contradict established science, but his use of experiments was extraordinary. He showed that when an artery was isolated by ligatures in the live animal, it did not contain air but blood. When he tied a hollow feather stem (canulla) into one of the arteries, it spurted out blood.[17] In other words, arteries contained blood as a normal condition, not only in disease, as Erasistratus thought. Observing blood in the arteries of the transparent mesentery gave him further support.[18] By opening the left ventricle in live animals, he found blood there, too. The whole left ventricular-arterial system contained blood, contrary to ingrained concepts, a substantial discovery. A major error tarnished the discovery, however. Since the right ventricle contained blood, how did it get to the left side? He did not know anything about the lesser circulation. He postulated that the heart had to force blood from the right to the left through invisible passages in the interventricular septum, but he hedged about the whole problem: he said pneuma and blood were in both ventricles, but there was more pneuma in the left. But what was pneuma supposed to be? Do we clarify the ancient words if we substitute oxygen for pneuma? That might be the solution. But what did he actually understand the word *pneuma,* or the Latin word *spiritus* to mean? Was it air or was it a hypothetical substance not clearly defined? It derived, he thought, from the liver as *spiritus naturalis* that, when combined with blood as *spiritus vitalis,* flowed from the left ventricle to the whole body, or was transformed into *"spiritus animalis"* in the brain.[19]

The theory of these three spirits was so persuasive that it survived more than thirteen hundred years after Galen's death. Only the discovery of blood circulation in the seventeenth century and the discovery of oxygen in the eighteenth put an end to the Galenic "spirits" and "pneuma." In the years of the Reformation in the sixteenth century the word *spirit* caused confusion and controversy, as it had multiple meanings in the contemporary Latin: enthusiasm, bravery, essence of liquor, and soul, or Spiritus Sanctus (Holy Spirit).

Further misconceptions of Galen were the pores of the interventricular septum and the idea that suppuration was necessary for wound healing. There were also many anatomical distortions because observations on animals were carried over to human conditions without restraint.[20] But what held the medical community spellbound for such a long time? Partly, it was due to the lack of human dissections and medical teaching institutions in the Roman Empire but also to the unsettled political situation of the Mediterranean and all of Europe. The final destruction of the only significant scientific center and library, in Alexandria, also had to do with it.

Allegedly, in 46 B.C. the library and the mouseion were already damaged when Julius Caesar laid siege. His invading ships were set on fire, which spread to the warehouses of the harbor and from there to the buildings of the institution. Yet most of the treasures of the library were spared. In the following centuries, however, substantial harm was suffered from time to time. Just a few years after Galen's death the suspicious new emperor Caracalla, to secure power, killed his brother and some twenty thousand other supporters in A.D. 211. Four years later Caracalla entered Alexandria, where he was criticized for his bloody deeds. As revenge he ordered all youth who could bear arms to be massacred.[21] Officials of the mouseion "were deprived of their revenues and those who were not natives of the country, were expelled," according to the historian Joseph Bidez.[22]

Two centuries after Galen, Alexandria came increasingly under the sway of Christian influence, especially after Constantine I converted to Christianity (A.D. 316) and developed the city into one of the most powerful bishoprics. Religious tensions soon surfaced over the Nicaean Council of A.D. 325, the role of the moderate faction of the Arians, and the demands of the radicals. Those different groups chose or deposed their bishops, sometimes with rough military force.[23] To confuse the situation further, large Jewish and pagan populations acted and counteracted against each other. One of those conflicts resulted in great damage to the mouseion. The overzealous bishop Theophilos took literally the decree of the emperor Theodosius I to destroy the heathen temples "throughout the whole world." He not only destroyed the Temple of Serapis but, in A.D. 390, also pillaged the library as another of the "pagan monuments."[24]

In the fourth, fifth, and sixth centuries, Greek intellectual influence waned because of frequent turmoil caused by invasions, warfare, and the struggle for survival everywhere in Europe and the Mediterranean basin. Alexandria lived on its reputation, while the Greco-Roman culture faded and the Christians grew stronger until the seventh century, when Muhammad's teachings took root in the Arab world and Alexandria suffered the grueling experience of a fourteen-month siege. When the Moslem chief general Amr took the city in A.D. 640, he could see for himself that its fame was not exaggerated when it was called second only to Rome. Amr duly reported to the khalif Omar about the four thousand palaces and the four hundred theaters and places of amusement in the city. In a letter he asked how he should handle the Royal Library because a philosopher had implored him to spare the valuable collection. Omar's answer was: "If those books contain the same doctrine as the Koran, they could be of no use, since the Koran does contain all the necessary truths. If they contain anything contrary to it, they ought to be destroyed."[25] So the scrolls were given as fuel to the four thousand public baths to supply fire for their "tepidariums."

The products of the first reign of reason in science went up in smoke. Some historians doubt this story, but the sad fact remains that all seven hundred thousand volumes of the Royal Library and the two hundred thousand copies next to the Serapis Temple disappeared. After centuries of disorder and military actions, not a single volume survives.

Later, the destruction and upheaval gave way to Islamic culture. In the vast area of Arabic dominance that stretched from Persia to southwest Europe, two centers developed into fountainheads of the natural sciences: Baghdad, not far from the site of ancient Babylon, and Cordoba in Spain. In Baghdad, bordering the Tigris River, the Arabs adopted the mathematical traditions of Hindu sages who were influenced by the Greeks and by the Babylonian priests who knew so much about calculation of stars and their movements.

At the end of the eighth century, a Hindu astronomer was invited to Baghdad and introduced Hindu numerals into Arabic mathematics. The works of Euclides and Ptolemy (the astronomer) were translated under the enlightened influence of Harun al-Rashid (786–809).[26] The numerals that were to supersede the Roman numerals originated in India, possibly in the third century B.C., when the Greeks under Alexander had contact with them. The symbol 0 (zero) was also introduced there where "the contemplation of an absolute void or nothingness characterizes native philosophy."[27] The complete Hindu-Arabic number system including the zero, which was not noted in Roman times, was introduced in Baghdad and spread along the trade routes to Europe from the ninth century on, but it gained recognition rather slowly. In the fourteenth century Florentine bankers were forbidden to use it, but the fact that its use was prohibited shows that they actually did take advantage of it, although Roman numerals were still used in government accounts as late as 1734 in France and on medical prescriptions in the twentieth century in central Europe.[28] The Hindu-Arabic numerals helped mathematical calculations, particularly multiplication and division, so difficult with the ancient symbols, and they made possible a numerical assessment of the universe.

But what did the Arabs contribute to medicine? With their bent toward mysticism, they explored alchemy (the word itself is of

Arabic origin) and consequently enhanced knowledge in chemistry with deeper insight into the nature of drugs and poisons. What they knew about the human body they received from ancient Greece and Rome. Under some of the well-educated caliphs, translation of Greek texts was fostered either from Syrian translations made in Roman imperial times or from original manuscripts or copies from Byzantium (present-day Istanbul, Turkey). Translation committees, chaired by respected scholars, were organized to enhance and speed up the work. Galen remained the main source of information with all his mistaken ideas about medicine. Although the Arabs contributed to clinical observation and to pharmacology, they did nothing in anatomy, physiology, or pathology. Dissections were made impossible by the strict rules of the Koran, prescribing in detail how to handle corpses.[29] None of the often-quoted Arabs introduced anything new in this line, except for a man barely ever mentioned—Ibn al-Nafis.

The introduction of his anatomy book gives due respect to the authorities: "We were held back from dissection by our respect for the law and our inborn compassion." But he notes, when describing the heart, "Between the two ventricles . . . there is absolutely no opening, for if there were, blood could enter into the place of spiritus, spoiling its composition. Dissection further refutes this assertion, for the partition between the two chambers is thicker than elsewhere." Al-Nafis was the first to arrive at the description of the lesser circulation: "The pores of the heart are closed at that point (the septum), its substance is tough, leaving no doubt that after refinement, the blood gets into the lungs by way of the vena arteriosa (artery-like vein = pulmonary artery), there to spread and combine with air, and the purified part still further refined, flows into the arteria venosa (vein-like artery = pulmonary vein) to reach the left ventricle." Today, of course, instead of the blood's "purified part still further refined," we would say oxygenated blood. Regardless, al-Nafis was the first to contradict Galen in respect to the interventricular septum and to describe the lesser circulation— discoveries that had to wait an additional three and a half centuries to be refound.[30]

But why was al-Nafis almost forgotten, while others without any original thoughts were quoted and praised all over the Arab world and Europe for a long time? At last a partial answer can be found in the political situation. Al-Nafis made his findings in Cairo just when the two major centers of Islamic culture and book production were lost to the sciences. Cordova fell to Castile in 1236, and Baghdad was taken by the Mongols in 1258 when some eight hundred thousand people were massacred in and around the city.[31] Also, al-Nafis did not give credit to Galen in every instance, whereas his teachings were followed almost to the letter by all scholars, so al-Nafis's lonely word did not stir any echo.

To the Arabs we owe the preservation of Greek philosophical thought, which spread mainly from Spain and Persia to medieval Europe. Many students gathered in those two intellectual centers to acquire polish and culture. A pope, Sylvester II (945–1003), brought the Arabic numerals to Europe from Spain, where he spent some years of his youth. He also learned there that the earth was not flat but spherical. He constructed a hemisphere to teach imaginary celestial circles and a sphere to show the planetary orbits. His contemporaries spread contradicting rumors: that the pope's knowledge came from the Devil himself, or that the pope was sent by God.[32]

After the unruly migrating groups settled in Europe in territories that became their countries and after the convulsions of the Crusades, the Mongol invasion, and the struggle for might between popes and emperors subsided, the citizenry in the towns finally had a chance to deal with more than mere survival. Stupendous cathedrals were built, and about eighty universities were founded between 1200 and the end of the Middle Ages. Although a few dissections were performed at a small number of universities (including Padua and Bologna), the teaching of medicine followed the trodden path of the ancients. Education consisted of honoring known doctrines and memorizing passages from books. It was probably an important way to convey thoughts as books were rare and expensive; students could not afford to have them at their disposal. Unfortunately, that method took a lot of time away from original thinking and, without experimentation, led to ready acceptance of ancient practices, explanations, and mistakes.

Despite the static atmosphere, slowly progressive tendencies started to surface parallel to urbanization and the decline of papal authority. But then catastrophe struck again: a devastating plague swept through Europe from 1343 to 1356, killing a fourth of the population. Teaching in schools and universities was disrupted, and local and general governmental organizations were faced with rising crime rates and corruption. Agricultural products could not reach the townships, and the whole economy was in shambles. To give an inkling of how life was affected, let us turn to contemporaries: "What shall I say?" wrote Petrarch to a friend. "Where shall I begin? Where shall I turn? Suffering everywhere. Terror everywhere. Oh my friend, would that I had never been born, or already died. The sick man lies miserably alone in his home, not one of his relatives dares to approach him. The priest himself is filled with dread as he hands him the sacraments. Children cry heartbreakingly to their parents, fathers and mothers to their sons and daughters, husbands and wives to each other. But all in vain."[33] Boccaccio wrote similar lines: "Those left alive are crazy with fear and in their terror have no thought but for themselves. . . . In this terrifying collapse, the laws of God and man have disappeared, everyone acts for himself."[34] The pandemic left Europe bewildered and much less devoted to religion than before. Didn't as many pious people die as rascals? And were prayers of any help?

After the confusion and fear for life faded, some promising innovations emerged that changed the course of history and the sciences. Henry the Navigator (1394–1460) organized an innovative institute at the southern corner of Portugal. He gathered mapmakers, mathematicians, and astronomers from wherever he could get them—regardless of race, nationality, or creed—to help captains of ships explore the secrets of the oceans. The mariners, in turn, reported to the scientists their findings about currents, winds, and their experiences along the shores of Africa. This knowledge reaped results some decades later with the circumnavigation of Africa and the discovery of America.

At the same time the spiritual horizons were widened by a technical invention: the first book was printed from movable type about 1453. Printing with carved wooden blocks was practiced before that time, but the blocks were difficult to make—and therefore limited to playing cards or a few pages—and the process was expensive and slow. With movable type hundreds of pages could reach anybody for a cheaper price, and the type could be used again and again for other texts. Learning and knowing were not the privilege of a few any longer. News and thoughts reached everybody, raised the aspirations of the people, and changed their views about their surroundings and the universe—and about themselves.

4

Renaissance: The Eye-Opener, 1450–1543

THE CONTROVERSIAL GENIUS OF Emperor Frederick II (1215–1250) broke the stifling practice of not daring or wanting to look into the human body. Originating in northern Europe, he was raised in Sicily, where there was still a large population of Arabs. Eager to know everything from all angles but not influenced by scholastic doctrines, Frederick absorbed all the languages that he encountered: Greek, Latin, Italian, Arabic, and German. In that melting pot, he developed a free spirit that made it possible for him to dare the unusual.[1] In his military campaigns and his own devastating encounter with the plague (which, as a rare exception, he survived), he must have become disgusted with the ignorance of the doctors. Since he wanted to make them more knowledgeable, in 1238 he ordered public dissections to be performed every five years at the medical school of Salerno (in southern Italy, which was under his command), and he decreed that no one should practice surgery without having studied anatomy for one year.[2] Because of continuous political unrest and wars, this innovative thought diffused rather slowly toward central and northern Italy. Yet an anatomy book was written by Mondino in Bologna in 1316 (on the basis of just two dissections), following basically the footsteps of Galen. Public dissections were performed during the fourteenth century in Padua, Genoa, and Ferrara.[3] The Venetian government made it a

33

duty in 1335 for the twelve doctors-surgeons to whom the Republic paid full salary, and for all licensed practitioners, to attend an annual course of anatomy that included dissection of corpses.[4]

Strangely enough, the painters and sculptors rather than the medical doctors showed an original interest in human anatomy, first of all in Florence. Toward the 1400s, Florence developed into the leading commercial center of Europe. Importation of wool from England, and silk and spices from the Orient brought in by a large merchant fleet through Pisa, served to spread the most beautifully designed and colored final products of textiles and furs over the known world. With some eighty banks the Florentines started the first detailed accounting system to keep track not only of their daily casual expenses or income but also of monies lent to princes, kings, and popes. Through their commerce with all of Europe, and with Constantinople in particular, Florentine scholars became acquainted with the original manuscripts of the ancient Greek philosophers, among them Plato and Aristotle. Classic Greek and Roman authors were studied extensively for their style and thoughts in that affluent society. Cosimo de' Medici, the most powerful banker of Florence, bought rare manuscripts from Greece and engaged forty-five copyists to transcribe those he was unable to buy. He wanted to obtain firsthand information about the philosophy of those ancient savants.[5] Cosimo tried to conduct internal as well as foreign policy to avoid perilous adventures such as wars. Consequently, under his leadership, and that of his son and grandson, between 1440 and 1490, Florence saw prosperity equal only to that of Venice.

The rich were eager to show their importance by building palaces and filling them with the most elaborate furniture, paintings, and sculpture. Artists were in high demand. As the models for artworks were ancient Greek and Roman statues, the ideal became the naked human body in its most appealing form. Medieval figures wrapped in heavy dresses were things of the past; likenesses of saints, even Jesus Christ himself, were dressed in scant garments. The study of the proportions of the body and its appearance became indispensable for a good artist. Piero della Francesca (1415–1492) wrote a book on perspective for painters. Leone Battista Alberti (1404–1472), in his treatise on painting, advised artists to draw human figures first nude, to give the limbs and body the proper proportions, and only afterwards paint their clothing. Donatello (1386–1466) was interested in anatomy, as his bronze plaque *The Anatomy of the Miser's Heart* attests. Luca Signorelli (1442–1524) had his favorite son stripped of his clothes after he became the victim of a violent death "and made drawings of the body so that he might always behold in this work . . . what Nature had given him and cruel Fortune had taken away."[6] Andrea del Castagno (1421–1457) made dissections, Antonio Pollaiuolo (1432–1498) flayed corpses to study their muscles, and Andrea del Verrocchio (1435–1488), who worked with Pollaiuolo and was apprenticed to Donatello, is also presumed to have studied anatomy.[7] The goal of those artists was to represent the human body with proportions and surface relief as realistically as possible and in aesthetic form to please the eye. This is how the most talented pupil of Verrocchio, Leonardo da Vinci (1452–1519), began. But as with everything else, he reached out further than his contemporaries.

Growing out of the fertile intellectual ground of Florence, Leonardo searched deeper and deeper into all human activities. He wanted to explore beyond the outlines of the muscles, their performance of physical work, the mechanism of breathing, of sneezing, of vomiting. He set the goal for himself to "describe what the soul is."[8] In one of the pages of his notes, he composed a preface for the planned book on anatomy. Here is the abbreviated version of a lengthier draft in his own words:

> This my depiction of the human body will be shown to you just as you had a real man before you. . . . It is necessary to make . . . anatomies, three of which you will need to acquire complete knowledge of the veins and arteries, destroying everything else with the utmost care; three others to acquire a knowledge of the membranes; three for the cords, muscle and ligaments; three for the bones and cartilages; and three for the anatomy of the bones which must be sawn through to demonstrate which are hollow and which not, which are medullary, which are spongy. . . . You must also make three of the female body in which there is a great mystery owing to the womb and its fetus. . . . Through my plan every part and every whole (region) will be made known to you . . . as if you had the same member in your hand and went on turning it gradually until you had a complete understanding of what you wish to know. . . . And might it so please our Creator that I be able to demonstrate the nature of man and his customs in the way that I describe his figure.[9]

Leonardo approached this vast task without indoctrination. As an artist he had no schooling in medicine. He did not belong to the Platonic Academy circle of Florence where the ideas of Plato and Aristotle (including the false medical ones) were taught and admired. He became acquainted with Galen and the Arabs only after he was well ahead of them in his own studies so he was not influenced by their thoughts. All medical writers of his time, indoctrinated in the universities, tried to tailor their text and logic to Galenic patterns. On the contrary, Leonardo's initial ignorance in medical matters enhanced his neutrality of judgment; it was an advantage rather than a drawback. When he researched something, he inspected it and depicted what he saw, then added his explanations, referring eventually to Galen but not necessarily accepting his views.

After his glorious days in Milan in the court of the Duke Sforza, Leonardo's artistic world crumbled. His large twenty-six-foot-high clay model of the equestrian statue of the duke's father, praised for its dynamic force and beauty, was ruined by invading troops in 1500 (Leonardo was forty-eight years of age at the time); the French archers used it for target shooting. His patron defeated, Leonardo left Milan. The engineering assignment of the Venetian Republic and then of Cesare Borgia in 1501–1502 compelled him to travel from town to town in central Italy. He was more interested in doing architectural and machinery design and in studying aerodynamics and flying and declined to be involved in painting.[10] But the mysterious Borgia prince, and rumors of his cruelty, were unnerving. The strangling of one of Leonardo's friends on the prince's orders was more than he could tolerate.[11] He left the prince and returned to Florence, the city of his youth. He took up painting again, completing an altar piece and the Mona Lisa. The Signoria (Council of the Republic) persuaded him to paint a mural for the town hall. He worked on it diligently, but it started to decay before it was finished because of his faulty experimental technique, employing oily pigments on the wall. The breathtaking, fierce battle scene is preserved for us only by the copy of a carton done by Rubens many decades later, but the carton itself also has disappeared. Interruptions at his working places and the changing of patrons due to uncontrollable political circumstances discouraged

Leonardo in his artistic career. He drifted away from painting and devoted more time to the sciences and specifically to anatomy.

His drawings of human anatomy, which he said derived from thirty dissections, are veritably superb. Many of them are quite accurate. The mastery of the drawings themselves would make the collection a memorable one, but the distinctive observations, the novel approaches in his studies, make it unique. He used running water or lime water during dissection.[12] In an inventory of equipment for his autopsies, he noted gloves, a change of shoes, and, for the first time ever, a magnifying glass in biological study.[13] He was systematically sawing through bones, which nobody had practiced before him, and that is how he correctly drew the double curve of the spinal column. He was first to illustrate the frontal and maxillary sinuses. The skeleton and the skull had started to show up in contemporary medical texts, but they were exceedingly poor and inaccurate representations—compared to Leonardo's drawings.

The drawings of muscles of limbs from all sides could have been of great help to a painter, but Leonardo went far beyond artistic goals. The explanation and illustrations of the intercostal muscles and the pectoralis and serratus as auxiliary muscles for breathing could be used in a modern textbook. He introduced two methodical innovations in his muscular studies. To see the correlation of different muscles to each other at the very same time, so that the superficial muscle should not cover the one deeper seated, he tied wires or strings to the insertions after he cut off the muscles themselves. In this way he was able to show the architecture of the crisscrossing of succeeding layers. Or he made cross sections of limbs and observed the nerves and vessels embedded between the muscles as they are now shown to surgeons in topographical anatomy books.

The abdomen and gastrointestinal tract were not his forte, yet the liver and spleen were drawn correctly in glaring contradiction to contemporary drawings, in which the liver was shown with five identical leaves posing as banana peels.[14] He was the first to draw pictures of the appendix—although he gave false explanation to its nature. The single compartment of the uterus with a fetus in situ was drawn realistically for the first time in history, whereas ancient writings quoted by everybody at the time spoke about two compartments of the uterus, some of five or even seven.[15] A fully developed placenta is not depicted; rather, cotyledons are shown facing the uterus all around. Possibly he projected animal findings into human conditions.

The erection of the penis was thought to be due to pressure by air, but Leonardo explained it by arterial blood.[16] A cross section of a female and male in the act of lovemaking is as cool and scientific as can be. The text underneath reads, "In this way ulcers and disease may result," a premonition of the contagiousness of syphilis described by Fracastoro some thirty years later.[17]

A giant innovation was presented in the nervous system. In those days it was thought that the intellectual process was located around the cerebral ventricles. But having only a vague guess of the ventricular system, the compartments were described and drawn as three lemon-sized cavities placed side by side, or behind each other. On the basis of his readings, this is how Leonardo drafted his first illustration, but during his dissections he found something very different. He thus decided to explore their proper shape and proportions. As an artist he used the "lost wax" method well known to sculptors: "Pour wax through the hole 'n' at the bottom of the base of the cranium before it is sawn through. Make two vents in the horns of the great ventricles and inject melted wax with a syringe. . . . Then when the wax has set, take away the brain and you will see the shape of the ventricles perfectly."[18] Although the wax cast was not quite perfect, it represented a vast improvement over the distorted imagery of the ancients. It was the first time that anybody filled any compartment of the body with material that, after taking its shape, became rigid, making it possible to remove the walls of the cavity to render it visible. It was, in other words, a precursor of corrosion preparations and encephalography, angiography, or contrast studies of any kind.

The function of the spinal cord was followed with a crude, but enlightening experiment: "The frog retains life for some hours when deprived of his head, heart and intestines. But if you prick the said nerve [spinal cord], it suddenly twitches and dies."[19]

The cranial nerves were described fairly well. Interested in optics, Leonardo dealt extensively with the eyes at several stages of his studies, although he followed the faulty concept that the lens was in the middle of the bulb, despite trials to secure the position of the slippery contents of the eyeball. In order to have a firmer grip, he embedded the eye in egg white and then boiled it with the entrapped eyeball before cutting through. Yet the lens dislocated from its original place toward the middle, and this is how he described it. But looking at that fine optical instrument, he could not resist jotting down the following: "Who would believe that so small a space could contain the images of all the Universe? What talent can avail to penetrate a nature such as this? What tongue will it be, that can unfold so great a wonder? Truly none. This it is that guides the human discourse to the considering of divine things."[20]

But of all of Leonardo's achievements, his studies of the cardio-vascular system are most impressive. His drawings of the outside of the heart are marvelous representations of the surface of the heart, not schematically primitive like the contemporary medical illustrations, but realistic and meticulous with the coronaries, the coronary vein, and (on the inside), the cordae, the papillary muscles, the "moderator band" (called septomarginal trabecula today), and the foramen ovale. When it comes to the valves and their function, we are astonished by his intellect, which penetrated to depths explored only later by others, when detailed knowledge had cleared the way from the rubble that blocked lucid, unobstructed vision. Showing his thinking about the heart and respiration, areas then burdened by false concepts, he stated: "It seems to me impossible that any amount of air whatsoever should be able to enter the heart through the trachea, for if we try to inflate the heart, we will be unable to blow any air out of it."[21]

To deal with the difficulties of explaining hemodynamics according to Galenic concepts of motion of blood—spiritus, air—he could not cope with all the suppositions about the function of the valves, and therefore he wrote in embarrassment: "Doubts of this sort are subtle and difficult to prove or clarify."[22] In order to get an answer to the confusing questions, he resorted to making a model to study the currents of blood, keeping in mind his studies with water currents.[23] He recommended: "Plaster mold to be blown with thin glass inside and then break it from head to foot. . . . But first pour was into the valve (aortic valve) of a bull's heart so that you may see the true shape of this valve."[24] Or as we would express today: make a wax cast of the inside of the aorta, then take the tissues away, surround the wax with plaster of Paris, pour the melted wax out of it, blow thin glass into the plaster mold, and finally break it from top to bottom from the glass. Leonardo showed his glass model in several drawings and even gave instruction to glue membranes to the inside of the model to simulate the valves.[25] Most likely, he drew the turbulent flow according to experiments performed with fine grass seeds in his glass model.[26] His streamlines are almost identical with the 1972 pulse duplication studies of Wieting, which were conducted in a glass model with the aid of ciné filming by investigators who knew nothing about Leonardo's studies of some five hundred years earlier.[27]

Dealing with the vascular system, Leonardo drew arteries and veins correctly many times, but sometimes incorrectly. For instance, he repeatedly drew the right pulmonary veins communicating with the inferior vena cava. On the other hand, his observation on arteriosclerosis leaps forward by centuries. In the hospital of Santa Maria Novella in Florence he was allowed to watch sick patients and perform autopsies. He described one day's experience: "An old man only a few hours before he died, told me that he had lived for one hundred years without experiencing any physical failure or weakness; and sitting there on the bed in the hospital . . . he passed from this life giving no sign of any accident. I dissected his body in order to understand the cause of so easy a death and I found that the blood in the arteries nourishing the heart and the rest of the body, had decomposed and dried up. In my examination of a two-year-old boy I found everything quite different."[28] In another passage he wrote: "With advancing age the blood vessels lose their straight course and become increasingly twisted and bent as well as thicker. The question arises why the vessels should become winding where they were straight previously, and why their walls should thicken to such extent as to hinder or prevent the flow of blood and whether without any actual disease this might in itself be the cause of death in old people. . . . These old people gradually are crumbling away and are using up their life in the absence of nourishment."[29]

All these precious passages and drawings were put down at random, strewn over each other in a disorderly array as study notes. Leonardo must have felt that he was advanced enough with them to set them in order because he wrote around 1507–1509: "Have your books on anatomy bound"; and in 1510: "This winter of 1510 I think I will finish all this anatomy."[30] He definitely wanted to publish a book on anatomy, but whether it was in a form presentable to printers is very doubtful.[31] In 1778, 779 drawings were reported, but how many were lost during the two and a half centuries since Leonardo's death cannot be guessed. At the end of the nineteenth century there were only six hundred recorded in Windsor Castle and some scattered in Milan, Leipzig, and Paris. It is not impossible that only the finished pages were set aside, separate from the sketches, or perhaps are hidden in a forgotten corner of a museum or private collection. Just a few years ago pages were found in a Madrid museum. Will other pages surface unexpectedly in other places?

Leonardo assigned great importance to his work. "Concerning the advantage which I would like to hand down to mankind I shall teach you a process of printing, and I ask you my successors not to let yourselves be turned aside by motives of jealousy from making such prints."[32] In typical Leonardesque fashion, he found the current printing techniques inadequate and designed an improved printing press. But how could a book have been printed without an organized text, well-labeled illustrations in finalized form, and full attention paid to the huge amount of work such a task would have required? Not only was the failure due to his frequent changes of residence and his diverse obligations but also to his inability to follow through on such an immense project.

His beautiful drawings, his original observations, his ingenious and novel techniques lay stashed away in unworthy hands and only infrequently were admired by artists unaware of their medical value. His reverse writing, which could be read only by use of a mirror, further hampered any attempt at easy reading. Several centuries passed before his work received recognition, and by that time his findings were rediscovered.

Was Leonardo's work a miscarriage of progress? Was it worthwhile since it did not influence medical thinking? Was it superfluous altogether, despite its great vistas and potentials? Leonardo's marvelous achievements are the outcome of an attitude diametrically opposed to that prevalent in the Middle Ages. Giving full credit to Leonardo's genius, it was not his thinking alone that broke away from previous paths and pointed in new directions. It was the manifestation of a trend that has brought us to much higher levels of knowledge—and several others took that same direction.

5

Results of a New Kind of Approach, 1543–1895

BY THE TIME OF Leonardo's death, Europe was aflame with the religious controversies started by Luther's Ninety-five Theses (1517) and with the claims of serfs and peasants for better living conditions and more rights. The newly found riches of America shifted commerce and banking away from the accustomed trading posts of the Mediterranean coast and central and northern Europe to the western shores of Europe. Many countries were left with failing economies. Moreover, the arrogance of the nobility and government officials, injustice, and increased taxation led to open confrontation with authorities.[1] People drifted away from submission to medieval ideas about right and wrong, truth or fallacy. But the triggering force was not the economic side of life alone. Hardship had been experienced many times previously without this outcome. The proliferation of books set heads spinning with new ideas.

Curiously enough, in the natural sciences the printing press first cramped rather than loosened knowledge. After the Bible (the first printed book), educated people turned to the ancient writers quoted by theologians. The philosophy of Plato and Aristotle generally conformed with the ethics of religious dogma, whether Catholic or Protestant. Just as the ancient philosophers were given credence in the question of ethics, they were consulted on other questions as well. The natural sciences were read in either the original Greek or Latin, and few dared to contradict them. As Aristotle was referred to in politics, aesthetics, ethics, even biology, Galen was regarded as the authority in medicine. Editions of Galen and commentaries on his works were in the mainstream of interest, and printing companies were eager to satisfy their customers with the latest and best versions of his voluminous deliberations. Of all European cities striving for supremacy in the new art of printing, Venice was the most active. The capital of a widespread maritime empire with its republican constitution, the center of free thinking, and academics independent from clerical oppression, it could boast of 150 printing presses in the first half of the sixteenth century, publishing hundreds of books every year.[2]

Publisher Giunta embarked on printing an updated Latin version of Galen's works. For this enterprise he invited several authors to participate in the preparation of the book, among them Andreas Vesalius, professor of surgery and anatomy of the Paduan medical faculty. Giunta had good reason to select the twenty-four-year-old professor for the task. Vesalius had come originally from Brussels, then through Paris to Padua just a few years earlier. He was already well respected not only for his medical knowledge but mainly for his skill in dissections and his insistence that uneducated men should not be allowed to perform the dissections. He was known to the faculty for his publications (*Tabulae anatomicae sex,* 1538; *Institutiones anatomicae,* 1538; *Letter on venesection,* 1538), for which some of the illustrations he himself drafted. Most of the text and illustrations followed Galen's descriptions (five lobes of the liver, etc.), although some deviated from them. As Vesalius encountered more differences between Galen and reality, he decided to go into depth with every single inch of the human body. Meanwhile, he prepared his section of the Giunta edition, which gave him the best opportunity to become acquainted with Galen's teachings— and errors. He relentlessly sought to know more about the body's construction. His public dissections were frequented not only by students and physicians but also by professors from other faculties, leading citizens of Padua and Venice, and even artists. At one presentation, more than five hundred attended, and all "stayed to the very end."[3] A judge of the criminal court provided bodies of executed criminals for him—even scheduling the time of execution most convenient for Vesalius to pursue his studies.[4]

Public dissections were performed in temporarily erected tents or wooden shacks. Permanent autopsy rooms were not available, and so Vesalius in his zeal for study would occasionally store parts of corpses in his bedroom, keeping them there for weeks for further examination.[5] He was even interested in peculiarities of people: overextension of joints, deformed heads of children shown in the circus, and performers who raised great weights with their teeth; he observed bones and tendons of beef on his dish at the dinner table.

He drew pictures of his findings during autopsies but also befriended a talented apprentice from Titian's studio, Johann Calcar, and persuaded him to make illustrations of the autopsy specimens. Other artists were also involved, most likely Titian's pupils, but none identified by name in the final book. This is a pity because the triumph of the final product is partially due to the superb illustrations. Incidentally, Vesalius did not know of Leonardo's drawings. Moreover, he did not have a high opinion of artists and occasionally had serious disagreements with them.

No matter where he looked, what he saw, or what he considered, everything connected with anatomy. Vesalius thought, breathed, and lived anatomy. In a short four years he wrote a book of seven hundred pages in large folio format with more than three hundred woodcut illustrations. A few of the drawings were by his own pen. A long chapter dealing with techniques and a substantial index were added to the *De humani corporis fabrica* in 1543.

Included in the work was a chapter on vivisection—physiological experiments, we would say. There is a notable description of the opening of the thorax: "The animal now all but suffocated by reason of the total collapse of the lungs. . . . So that life may in some measure be restored to the animal, you must attempt an opening in the trunk of the trachea and pass into it a tube of rush or reed and you must blow into this, so that the lung may expand and the animal draw breath after fashion; for at a light breath the lung in this living animal will swell to the size of the cavity of the thorax and the heart take strength afresh and exhibit a great variety of motion. . . . None of my discoveries in anatomy pleases me more."[6]

Vesalius decided to give the manuscript to the printing shop of his personal friend Andreas Oporinus of Basel, Switzerland, because there he could supervise the work of printers (as a matter of fact he spent six months there for that purpose). The woodcuts by several artists were carried from Padua through Alpine passes on the backs of mules so that the Basel printers could get the correct illustrations, which were best produced in Italy.[7]

The reader became convinced of the truth of every line written by Vesalius because the totally uncommitted observations were persuasive. There was no guessing, no fantasy substituting for reality, no fleeting remarks on anything.[8] Many previously held beliefs were criticized, or newly discovered details were described: menisci in joints, distinction of grey and white matter in the brain, the fornix, and the septum pellucidum. It was clarified that the uterus contains only one cavity (not two or seven) and that the liver does not have five separate lobes (as was taught up to his time). Incidentally, Vesalius compared the liver and other organs in different animal species with those observed in humans. Galen's statement that there is a bone in the heart and Aristotle's "third ventricle" in the cardiac septum were refuted.[9] Vesalius paid special attention to the septum because, according to Galenic teachings, blood seeped through its "pores" from the right to the left ventricle. "None of its pits," wrote Vesalius, "at least insofar as can be ascertained by the senses, penetrate from the right ventricle into the left. Thus we are compelled to astonishment at the industry of the Creator who causes the blood to sweat from the right ventricle into the left through passages which escape our sight."[10] A praiseworthy observation—only he should not have mentioned the Creator in a somewhat mocking tone in an age boiling with religious fervor.

The statement opposed Galen's view, and it was not the only criticism. As a matter of fact, Vesalius found that in more than two hundred instances he had to refute Galen's opinion.[11] It was not only the novelty of newly found structures and false ones properly corrected that created a stir but it was the novelty of approach that heralded a totally changed attitude toward investigations of the human body.

He felt the boldness of his undertaking, but with unshakable self-confidence he did not doubt the truth of his findings. One of the woodcuts of the *Fabrica,* a skeleton, is leaning on a block that bears the inscription: "The genius lives, the rest are dead." He dedicated the book to the emperor Charles V, stating bluntly: "I am aware that by reason of my age—I am at present 28 years old—my efforts will have little authority and that because of my frequent indication of the falsity of Galen's teachings, they will find little shelter from attacks. . . . Various schemes in defense of Galen will be boldly invented, unless these books appear with the auspicious commendation and great patronage of some divine power. They cannot be more safely sheltered or more splendidly adorned than by the imperishable name of the great and invincible Emperor, the divine Charles."[12]

In the same year of 1543, another book also appeared on the bookshelves in Europe, *On the Revolutions of the Heavenly Orbs,* by Copernicus, the Polish astronomer. The ancient world of Aristotle, Ptolemy, and Galen—which had dominated the world of thinking for more than fifteen hundred years—had to give way to new notions.

It was probably a reflection of favorable acceptance of the book by the emperor that Vesalius was summoned (or invited) to serve His Majesty as physician. This raised the jealousy of other physicians of the imperial court to whom it seemed offensive to see such a young man as a rival, even though he already had become famous by his book. Gossip and intrigue immediately arose against him. Rumors and attacks of Galenists piled up, and it appears that withdrawal from his assignment as the emperor's physician was not possible. In his depressed mood, he threw his voluminous medical notes into the fire and vowed never again to participate in scientific research, an act he later bitterly regretted.

The next years were spent in following the emperor on military campaigns, conferences, consulting, and participating in the treatment of high officials. He was first to diagnose a thoracic aneurysm, to treat a thoracic abscess by puncturing it, and to remove successfully a cancerous breast.[13] Occasionally, he had the chance to perform an autopsy to establish the cause of death, which led to pathological observations.[14] He also had to devote some time to defending his findings against opponents, among them a previous professor, Jacobus Sylvius, who went so far as to write a pamphlet against him in which he exclaimed: "I implore his Imperial Majesty to punish severely as he deserves, this monster, this worst example of ignorance, ingratitude, arrogance and impiety, to suppress him so that he may not poison the rest of Europe with his pestilential breath."[15]

The rude language was repugnant enough to readers that it did not harm Vesalius unduly, yet it must be noted that he himself irritated his opponents. About the Galenic "bone in the heart," he wrote: "Let us put aside this sort of imagining of men and let us condemn their stupidity."[16] About sesamoids (to which magic powers were ascribed), he said: "I leave this for the discussion of the theologians. . . . It is better known to superstitious men, than to students of anatomy."[17] And about the professors of anatomy he offered his most severe criticism: "The deplorable division of art of treatment induced into the schools that detestable procedure by which usually some conduct the dissections of the human body and others present the account of its parts, the latter like jackdaws aloft in their high chair with egregious arrogance croaking things they never investigated but merely committed to memory from the books of others."[18]

Years passed in bickering about his findings; nevertheless, the book was a great success. So great, indeed, that Giovanni Battista Canano (1515–1579), one of the first to describe the venous valves and muscles (1541), withdrew his 1541 treatise and did not pursue further work in anatomy. Some others were not so sensitive, as shown by several plagiaristic publications all over Europe, in which both text and illustrations were pirated.[19]

Meanwhile, Vesalius prepared the second edition of the book for publication in 1555, leaving aside the polemics and imprudent remarks that he had directed in his youthful brusqueness toward the clergy. He described some new findings: the human placenta, the corpora lutea, the proper presentation of sesamoids, and others.[20] Most noteworthy, his increased attention was given to the septum of the heart: "I have no knowledge that even the smallest amount of blood can be taken through the substance of the septum from the right ventricle to the left," and "the reason for the difference in thickness of the parts constituting the right ventricle and the left must be otherwise than for the materials contained in the ventricles. Many things present themselves here that call into doubt the ordinary conclusion of anatomists, but it would take too long to consider them and I have decided not to alter my account piecemeal—although at the same time I am far from satisfied."[21]

One wonders how far he could have gone given time. He did not know about the opinion of the Arab al-Nafis (see chapter 3) in this matter. Certainly, the question of "porosity" of the septum bothered Vesalius for a long time. As he dissected corpses in his student years in Paris, it is most likely that the Spaniard Miguel Servede (latinized Servetus), working with him, learned of his doubts. Servede was not a great experimenter; rather, he was interested in religious polemics. Buried between religious passages, he wrote: "Communication between the two ventricles does not take place across the tissue in the center of the heart as is generally believed but . . . through the right ventricle after it has pumped the purified blood through its long trip toward the lungs. In the lungs it is transformed and turned red. . . . The central partition plays no role in this communication or in the transformation of the blood, for it contains no blood vessels."[22] In 1555 Servede was sent to the stake in Geneva by Calvin and his followers, and most of his books were burned with him.

The same observation on the septum and the pulmonary circulation was published in 1559 in Venice by Realdo Colombo, a student of Vesalius in Padua who inherited his chair of anatomy for a few years.[23] Did Vesalius see the books of Servede or Colombo? There is no indication in his scripts.

Meanwhile, Vesalius was busy with his princely commitments. Removed from the mainstream of scientific activities of Padua and Bologna, he did not seem fully aware of what was going on in the world of science—until he received a book from Fallopius, professor in Padua (1523–1562).[24] Here was a work of a superior observer of tiny but important things: for example, the vestibular aqueduct, the osseous cochlea, the chorda tympani, details of the ocular muscles and nerves, the glossopharyngeal nerve, and the uterine tube (Fallopian tube). Fallopius corrected some mistakes of Vesalius, including the belief that the cerebral arteries ended in the sinuses.[25] Vesalius immediately wrote a lengthy reply to Fallopius in which he expressed nostalgic emotions of "that extremely pleasant life in which he took part in Italy, the real home of talent."[26] The letter never reached Fallopius, who died in 1562. Vesalius harbored a desire to return to Padua. Finally, in 1564, he received permission from Emperor Philip II to leave Spain with the stipulation that he first undertake a journey of pilgrimage to Jerusalem.

While different suppositions try to explain this journey, the most likely is the version of Ambroise Paré, the famous French surgeon (1510–1590) who knew Vesalius personally. According to Paré, Vesalius performed an autopsy on a Spanish noblewoman, and during the course of the dissection, the relatives, who were standing by, presumed to have seen the heart moving. Immediately, an accusation was levied against Vesalius by the Inquisition. His imprudent remarks on "theologians" in the first edition of the *Fabrica* certainly did not endear him. The passage of the book where he described how he carried "the still pulsating heart with the lung and the rest of the viscera" of a recently quartered criminal for examination must have served to incriminate him. But his many services at court worked in his favor, and he was permitted to leave.[27]

On the way to Jerusalem, he stopped in Venice, where the *Signoria* (government) appointed him for the second time to his old, now vacant chair of anatomy in Padua University.[28] Everything seemed to have turned out well for Vesalius. Fate, however, made a nasty twist. On the way back toward Venice from Jerusalem, the ship full of pilgrims had to struggle in a stormy sea for more than a month. Many people died, and Vesalius also became sick. He was put ashore on a small island near the Greek mainland. He passed away there alone in the midst of fishermen and peasants who did not have the faintest idea who the stranger was.[29]

In the same year (1564) a book was written in Rome by Bartolommeo Eustachio (1520–1574) in which, among other things, he described the pharyngotympanic tube, the modiolus in the cochlea, the musculus tensor tympani, and the stapedius muscle, and he first mentioned the suprarenals.[30] The book, however, was not published for another 150 years (1714). We do not know why. The chair of anatomy in Padua went to Fabrizio d'Aquapendente in 1565. He did extensive research in comparative embryology and wrote a small monograph on the valves of veins, both of which profoundly influenced his later-famous pupil William Harvey. Many other followers of Vesalius have contributed to the study of anatomy using his method: sound observation, disregard for dictum of authorities, and reasoning rather than speculation. It was Vesalius—with his intensity, his brash youthful force, his unrelenting faith in his working logistics—who created a new approach to scientific inquiry and pointed out the appropriate direction. He was the consequence and the originator of a scientific trend: to want to perceive reality without theory. The practice of personal observation exerted profound influence upon the contemporary minds, resulting in a series of discoveries that enriched the knowledge of the body. Yet these represented only an extension of the Vesalian concept—until unexpectedly a new dimension of a different nature appeared on the scene at the beginning of the seventeenth century: the extension of our visual capability, the very first entrance of technology to science.

Galileo noted in 1623: "News arrived at Venice . . . that a Dutchman had presented to Count Maurice of Nassau a glass by means of which one could see distant things as clearly as if they were near . . . the Dutchman . . . handling by chance different forms of glasses, looked . . . through two of them, one convex, the other concave . . . and noted the unexpected result."[31] Galileo, exuberant, optimistic in his expectations, immediately saw the gain that magnification of objects could bring to his science—and pocket.[32] When the senators and university professors looked into the device he had put together just a few days after the news, at the top of the Venice Campanile, and saw the ships on the horizon two hours before they became visible with the naked eye, Galileo knew his battle for fame and money had been won. In addition to his prime interest, the stars, he could not pass up the opportunity of directing his instrument to closer objects. According to a contemporary report, with his "occhialino" (microscope) he "has seen flies which look as big as a lamb."[33]

His magnifying instrument had a grave limitation, however: to enlarge objects nearby, the observer had to pull out the eye lens from the objective to two to three feet.[34] Microscopes of acceptable dimensions were produced some years later, and after the 1650s they were accepted by interested amateurs who looked at anything they could put their hands on. Followers of Cromwell snarled at the "virtuosi" that they "had an excellent faculty of magnifying a louse and diminishing the Commonwealth."[35] But serious subjects were also investigated with the microscope.

Malpighi in Italy made a momentous discovery of blood flow through capillaries that had evaded the scrutiny of Harvey. Robert Hooke made observations on plants and animals, following in the footsteps of Christopher Wren, the architect of St. Paul's Cathedral who also discovered the "Circle of Willis" and performed the first intravenous injection for pharmacological study.[36] Hooke was the first to coin the concept of "cell" in his study of plants. Loewenhoek described red blood cells in 1673 with the aid of his primitive single-lens microscope; the others used compound microscopes with two lenses. The grinding of lenses was cumbersome, however, and the assembly of the parts was difficult. The resulting products were not always of high quality, and the microscopical achievements of the 1660s and 1670s were not followed by substantial improvements for two centuries.

The leading trends in arts came from Italy, and so it was with the sciences. It is not surprising that anatomy experienced a fresh breeze from the same corner. Morgagni (1682–1771), at the young age of twenty-five years, became professor of theoretical medicine, then professor of anatomy in Padua. In the ensuing decades he made meticulous notes on dissected corpses. This was not unique since others before him had done the same. What was unusual was that he connected the clinical histories with his observations on the autopsy table and related those to other similar cases. His clinical experiences of his younger years and his broad knowledge of general medicine were added to his familiarity with normal anatomy, "the torch of pathological anatomy."[37] The unified view of the sick but still living person and the manifestation of disease at autopsy clarified many random findings. Although he respected the microscope, he was fully aware of its contemporary limitations: chromatic aberration cast all kinds of colored halos around the objects to be observed, and spherical aberration resulted in blurring images. Even decades later Bichat wrote: "If one watches in the dimness, everybody sees according to his taste, following its effects on him."[38]

Cautious man that he was, Morgagni put down his observations of seven hundred cases after a lifetime. He published *De sedibus et causeis morborum* in 1761, when he was already seventy-nine years of age. The work was a gold mine of treasures. To quote a few, he described the heart in angina and endocarditis; he recognized the "polyps" in the heart as postmortem clots; he related apoplexy to vascular changes in the brain; and he described diverse manifestations of syphilis, stages of pneumonia, cirrhosis of the liver, acute yellow atrophy, calculi in various locations, and tumors of diverse origin.

Many able investigators followed Morgagni's example up to the mid-nineteenth century, and a large volume of knowledge had been collected about the exact location of diseases and their appearances in organs. Old concepts of humors were still alive, however; Rokitansky, the leading pathologist in Vienna who allegedly performed thirty thousand autopsies during his active years, talked about "krasis," a contemporary form of Hippocratic humors. But as it happens frequently in the history of the sciences, some years and some places trigger substantial innovations because certain factors conglomerate then and there. This is what happened in Berlin in the 1830s. It was not the metropolis it is now, but much smaller, so that people of similar interests knew and influenced each other. Humboldt was there, as was the naturalist Richard Brown, who described the nucleus of the cell in 1832, and there was a host of young men full of ideas in Johannes Mueller's physiology institute. Microscopes based on the design of J. J. Lister (the father of the "antiseptic Lister") appeared, which eliminated the hitherto disturbing chromatic and spherical aberrations, allowing more accurate observation of details. It is said that Schleiden and Schwann at a "coffee time discussion" took up the concept that the cell, a miniature entity well circumscribed in the living organism, represented the unit upon which life depends.[39] Schleiden put the thought on paper about plants, followed by Schwann, who extended it to animal tissues (1837). This was such a persuasive notion that Professor Mueller sat down immediately and wrote a publication about the construction of tumors based on the progressive cell theory.[40] Young Rudolf Virchow (1821–1902), who happened to be in Mueller's laboratory at that time, took up the hint of the importance of the cell and moved it to the forefront of investigations. Without the improved microscopes, none of them would have been able to reach their advanced conclusions.[41]

In the following years Virchow showed that the cells are reproduced by division of their nuclei and that their appearance changes markedly in disease. He put the emphasis in disease process on the study of the cell, as carrier of pathological changes—well defined and well demonstrable—not on "humors." Virchow gave the first description of leukemia, thrombosis, and embolism, the definition of fatty degeneration, cloudy swelling, and amyloid change—many new things that moved pathology from inspection with the naked eye to microscopic dimension. His most talented pupil, Cohnheim, further extended his master's somewhat static views into dynamic experimental terrain.[42] In the ensuing decades the microscope was improved from magnifying powers of hundreds to thousands with the help of the Italian Amici and the German Abbe.[43] This helped to identify bacteria, another territory to explain diseases by visualization. Oddly enough, Virchow was skeptical about bacteriology; he considered social backwardness equally important to explain diseases (which is, of course, true), and he did not support hand washing and the theories of Semmelweis. Nevertheless, he put the cell in the center to explain diseases and, in doing so, he created pathology, as we now know the specialty.[44]

By the end of the nineteenth century most diseases were well described in detail on the autopsy table as well as in microscope. There was only one painful limitation: explanation of the living was still based on palpating, listening, and studying case histories— all very important, yet lacking visual confirmation. Because scientific minds were craving to see the inside of the living body, anything leading to seeing beyond the surface earned immediate success. After Helmholz described the ophthalmoscope in 1851, it was instantly caught up by the German von Grafe and the Dutch Donders and Snellen, and they built the specialty of ophthalmology. By 1855 Manuel Garcia, the singing teacher, made use of two mirrors, this time looking into his own larynx to watch the movements of the vocal cords. The Bohemian Czermak and the Viennese Turck both jumped on the idea (not knowing of each other) and developed laryngoscopy into such a success that their hurt vanity induced them to wage a fierce polemic battle for priority.[45]

Longing to look into the live body led Claude Bernard to daydreaming when he jotted down in his laboratory logbook: "One ought to devise an apparatus to watch a chick develop in an egg and be able to experiment on it without changing the conditions for its development. . . . It would be useful to construct a microscope examining living phenomena."[46] Paul Ehrlich tried to catch manifestations of life with methylene blue, staining the nervous system in vivo: "The staining of the dead gives us only anatomical clarification of architectural tissues. . . . If one wants to know about their function, one has to stain the normal tissues in the height of their activity."[47]

A new technique was needed to open up new possibilities, which only the basic sciences could have provided. But they remained silent. A. A. Michelson, the famous physicist and later Nobelist whose experiments guided Einstein to the relativity theory, observed when addressing the dedication of the Physics Laboratory of the University of Chicago: "The more important fundamental laws and facts of physical science have all been discovered, and these are now so firmly established, that the possibility of their ever being supplanted in consequence of new discoveries is exceedingly remote." He added sarcastically, "Our future discoveries must be looked for in the sixth place of decimal."[48]

The calendar recorded the year 1894.

6

First Look into the Living Human Body, 1895–1913

DESPITE MICHELSON'S discouraging prediction about the future of exploration in physics—which almost amounted to a declaration that the territory was without perspectives—some young and not-so-young physicists ventured to play with new ideas.

In 1895, Marconi, only twenty years old and a student at Bologna University, read in a scientific journal in his native Italy about the electric wave experiments of Hertz, who proved that electrical forces could jump over from one coil to another in air, without immediate contact.[1] Marconi could increase the few centimeters of Hertz and reach a distance of two kilometers with a large antenna. He conceived the idea that he could send messages with this kind of device, a "wireless telegraph." Thus, the concept of radio transmission was born.

At the same time a much older physicist, Roentgen (Röntgen), in his fiftieth year became interested in cathode rays. He was not the only one to become infatuated with those rays—whatever they were. It started with Plucker and Hittorf in Germany, who in the late 1860s had taken up the task of studying the conductivity of electricity in rarified gases. They observed a fluorescent light on the glass wall of the discharge tube opposite the cathode and noted that those "rays" emanating from the cathode traveled in a straight line.[2] Crookes in England took up the experiments, and during his studies he recognized that the cathode rays could be deflected by a magnet; thus, according to Faraday's rule, the rays had to consist of negatively charged particles.[3] "We seem at length to have within our grasp and obedient to our control," wrote Crookes, "the little indivisible particles which with good warrant are supposed to constitute the physical basis of the Universe. . . . I venture to think that the greatest scientific problems of the future will find their solution in this Border Land and even beyond; here . . . lie Ultimate Realities subtle, far-reaching, wonderful."[4] He thought the cathode rays were negatively charged molecules; nobody at that time knew about electrons—the atom was the ultimate indivisible particle of matter. The problem was the interpretation of these rays: the German scientists thought they represented electromagnetic waves like light; the English, influenced by Crookes, held that they were corpuscular in nature.

The difference of opinions let the imagination fly high. The physics laboratories with all their electrical coils, magnets, photographic cameras, condensers, and other instruments were buzzing with activity. In Philadelphia, for example, when Goodspeed found that in his experiments with cathode rays a photographic plate fogged in an undesirable way, he discarded the plate on a heap of other unusable products (1890); years later he realized that he had thrown away a gem. Likewise, Crookes in London complained about photographic plates that had to be returned to the manufacturer, as they were "very badly fogged."[5] William Thomson, who later was knighted for his research to become Lord Kelvin, read a paper in the Royal Society dealing with the velocity of cathode rays.[6]

The electromagnetic theory of light was proven experimentally by Hertz, who also became interested in cathode rays. Working on discharge tubes with his assistant Lenard, he observed different cathode rays "which can be differentiated from one another by their production of phosphorescence, by their absorption and by their deflection of a magnet."[7] Hertz concluded that they must be rays rather than particles because they could pass through a very thin foil of gold or aluminum; particles would have been unable to do that.[8] Hertz did not have the opportunity to pursue his experiments with so many new findings, for he came down with a malignant tumor, causing excruciating pain. Despite several surgical interventions, he expired at the beginning of 1894.[9]

After Hertz's demise, Lenard continued the experiments with cathode rays, with two important findings: the absorption of those rays depends on the degree of rarefaction of the discharge apparatus; and at a distance of eight centimeters a fluorescent screen held in front of the tube remained completely dark.[10] Besides his experiments, Lenard took charge of a three-volume edition of the works of Hertz. He also accepted an invitation to another university, which he abandoned after finding out that there was no possibility to work scientifically. The year 1895 consequently represented a total waste for his experimental goals.

That was the year that Roentgen developed an ever-increasing fascination with cathode rays. The newly elected dean of Würzburg University, he was a well-respected scientist in the community of physicists, on the grounds of his research about the influence of pressure upon various physical properties of different liquids and solid materials and the compressibility of liquids, and on investigations of magnetic forces in a dielectric when moved between two electrically charged plates of a condenser.[11] Toward the end of 1895, he spent more and more time with cathode rays. He collected tubes of the Hittorf, Crookes, and Lenard types of construction; and he repeated the experiments of Hertz and Lenard.

On November 8, 1895, while passing the current through his tube, Roentgen observed a faint light coming from a bench in the dark laboratory room, where only the cathode rays should have been visible. That other light was approximately one meter away from the tube and the gleam of the cathode rays. He stopped the discharge and in the total darkness lit a match to see where the light originated from. It was a small screen of barium platinum cyanide. He checked thoroughly and could find no light coming from the outside. He discharged the tube again, and as before the faint greenish clouds again showed their ever-moving whirls on the screen.[12] This little fata morgana must have come somehow or other from the tube. But cathode rays did not go that far out of the tube. What was it then? Roentgen moved the screen further and further away, but the light still showed up.

He could not tear himself away from the riddle. He lived in the same building with the laboratory, so Mrs. Roentgen sent for him to join her at dinner. He finally came but was speechless, and immediately after he had finished eating, he rushed back to the laboratory. Questions rose one after another to be answered. A couple of days later, when one of his best friends asked him what all that busy running and absentmindedness were about, he could only respond: "I have discovered something interesting, but I do not know whether or not my observations are correct."[13]

Holding the barium platinum cyanide screen in front of the discharge tube, he could see it light up, even when he inserted as a barrier one thousand pages or thick blocks of wood, sheets of hard rubber, or glass. All were "transparent" unless the glass contained lead, and then it became much less transparent. He noted that if he held "the hand between the discharge apparatus and the screen, one sees the darker shadows of the bones within a much fainter shadow picture of the hand itself."[14] Water, carbon, several liquids, even copper, silver, lead, gold, and platinum let rays through—"but only if the plates were not too thick." The experiments with these materials led to the conclusion that "transparency depends upon their density."[15] But why had those rays never been seen before, recorded, reported, perceived by anybody? It came to his attention that photographic plates are sensitive to the rays that he could name only with the letter accepted in mathematics for the unknown: the sign X.

But what were these X rays, and how did they differ from the cathode rays? If they were similar to light, they could be refracted; however, with prisms of glass, hard rubber, or aluminum this was not possible. He tried pulverized material that reflects light in different directions—but the X rays did not show any reflection. Air absorbed X rays to a much lesser extent than it did cathode rays. Furthermore, X rays could not be deflected by a magnet as could cathode rays; consequently, they could not possibly be identical with them. In the course of his feverish investigations of a few weeks, the only conclusion he was able to make was that "X-rays are not identical with cathode rays, but . . . they are produced by cathode rays," and that although some kind of relation seemed to exist between the new rays and light rays, the two behaved entirely differently.[16] Knowing that he had found something unheard of and important, he hurried to the secretary of the Würzburg Physical-Medical Society with his manuscript titled "A New Kind of Rays: A Preliminary Communication."

The secretary, just about ready to close the last issue of the *Proceedings,* read it on that very day and deemed it important enough to squeeze into the last nine pages of the last issue of 1895. On New Year's Day, Roentgen had his reprints at hand and was able to send them with X-ray photographs to leading physicists of Switzerland, Germany, France, and elsewhere. One of them, the professor of physics in Vienna, Franz Exner, was having a party in his home, and he showed the photographs of his good friend Roentgen to his guests, amongst them a colleague from Prague. The guest was so intrigued that he asked Exner to lend him the photographs, which he showed the next day to his father, who happened to be the editor of one of the leading papers in Vienna. No time was wasted; the January 5 Sunday issue of the *Presse* carried an enthusiastic article on the front page, indicating that diagnosis of diseases could be made and injuries of bones "without the flesh" could be photographed. The *London Daily Chronicle* took it up the next day (through cablegram), and within the short period of a single week the leading medical journals of the United States, England, France, and Italy carried articles about the new discovery. Every laboratory started to take photographs with the Rumkorf coil, Crookes tube, and photographic plates they all had had at hand for years.

The speed of the publication process is stunning. The first phase of communication, the description of findings, was rapid to begin with. For Harvey it took twelve years to put his experiments into writing, for Copernicus even more. One could argue that those experiences were centuries away. But let us turn to the nineteenth century, to Roentgen's century. How about Darwin? Only when Wallace was ready to announce his similar results and upon the coaxing and pressure of friends did Darwin finally publish his work. Semmelweis waited for years before he announced his observations on contamination in childbed fever. The second phase of publishing is the editing and printing process. In our days of efficiency and computerized publication, it takes an average of three to six months to have data printed. Roentgen's paper was printed in days. It was the fascination with the finding that did it. To see the inside of the living body—bones never seen before, except on the autopsy table—was unheard of. And the news not only affected the editor but everybody who heard about it. Like a tornado, the news swept through the scene, leaving a rubble of old notions and the terrain ready for building everything anew from scratch.

The worldwide acclaim was such that the German emperor Wilhelm II invited Roentgen to Berlin to demonstrate his photographs, which he did on January 13, 1896. Ten days later he gave a talk to the Würzburg Medical Society and took a photograph of the hand of von Koelliker, the famous anatomist. Everyone was impressed, and Koelliker proposed that the X rays should be called Roentgen rays, and this is how the rays are still known in German-speaking countries. All over the world Roentgen was congratulated, and everybody expressed high hopes about the rays that would finally let human vision penetrate through the skin and see disease, never before perceived.

Only one person did not rejoice: Lenard. Hadn't he made important contributions to clarify some of the questions with cathode rays? Hadn't he sent Roentgen the address of the manufacturer who assembled his tubes? Those rays that evaded him but gave Roentgen the crown of success—those rays he never called anything but "high frequency radiation," not even after he was awarded the Nobel Prize in 1905 for his cathode ray investigations. But why didn't Lenard and the other equally astute physicists dealing with cathode rays discover X rays? Perhaps the vacuum pressure in their tubes was not low enough, or perhaps the voltage they applied was not high enough, but probably they simply concentrated too much on cathode rays; they could think of nothing else, even if they saw unexplainable things like fogged photographic plates or the effect upon electrified bodies at a distance.

In science as in everything, if a door opens upon an unknown interesting area, people will stream through the gate pushing each other, trying to be the first to look at the territory, thrilling, never seen before. Roentgen opened the door and everybody rushed in: not physicists alone (although the discovery was related to physics), but laymen, electricians, newspaper reporters, medical doctors—everyone wanted to look at the miracle. And as a credit to the human mind, they all saw the fabulous potential of seeing inside the body, the everyday normal as well as the diseased. And it was not the twentieth century with its sophisticated radio communications, TV potentials, and video display—it was still the nineteenth century. Yet news spread in days; fantasy soared in seconds. Every hour new angles of physical properties of the new rays were examined. New medical information had been checked all over the scientifically interested world. The enthusiasm to see medically important processes was such that within a short year more than one thousand articles and forty-nine books were published about the developments. Between 1896 and 1901 about eight thousand X-ray films were taken at the Massachusetts General Hospital on three thousand patients.[17]

Still, the nature of X rays was mysterious. When, in April 1896, a reporter of *McClure's Magazine* asked Roentgen for his thoughts upon seeing the unexplained light on the painted cardboard, he answered: "I did not think, I investigated." Then the reporter asked: "Is it light?"—"No."—"Is it electricity?"—"Not in any known form."—"What is it?"—"I do not know."[18] Yet in 1896 and 1897 Roentgen published some further observations, and for another fifteen years nothing more of importance was discovered about the nature of X rays.

Edison, ever eager to pursue practical angles, thought he could improve the efficiency of Roentgen's original screen. He did. He hired a throng of chemists to work on this project. He and his team set out to check chemical compounds, and after having investigated eighty-five hundred compounds in three months, he came up with calcium tungstate, six times more brilliant than barium platinum cyanide. The chemists working with him contracted severe burns on their fingers as they checked the brilliance of the experimental screens by looking at their hands' shadows on the fluorescent screen. Edison designed the fluoroscopic device that Roentgen himself used in his experiments. Already within the first year of Roentgen's discovery, stereoscopic images were shown by Elihu Thomson; Trowbridge recommended immersing the X-ray tubes in oil (to prevent ever-menacing overheating) and the use of the rotating anode envisioned by Wood.[19] Yet the tube's performance was unpredictable. The gas contained in it changed in amount, and the degree of vacuum varied; consequently, the quality of the X rays produced fluctuated, not to mention the obstacle of the tube's blowing up at the most crucial moments.

The shortcomings of the "gas tube" plagued medical application, and the long exposure times were embarrassing. The well-known roentgenogram of Mrs. Roentgen's hand was exposed approximately for fifteen minutes, and a picture of the lumbar spine required more than an hour.[20] The gastrointestinal tract with its wormlike whirlings, the heart movements with pulsatile rush, even breathing made images smudgy. Nothing that moved had the chance of being depicted properly: only the organs or tissues that did not move—the bones. Most important, pathological bone conditions were described within the first decade of roentgenologic activities: fractures, osteomyelitis, tumors, and the development of bones in children—all could be seen by the surgeon for the first time.[21] Alban Koehler's groundbreaking *Borderlands of the Normal and Early Pathology in Skeletel Roentgenology* (1905) in that short time pinned down those specifics that represent life and disease in bone. So thorough was his treatment of the subject that even now the book, somewhat amplified, is found in every radiologist's office.

The presence of bones in the fetus induced obstetricians to try to visualize them in utero. The first pioneers were E. P. Davis in Philadelphia and H. Varnier with A. Pinard in Paris, who succeeded in showing fetuses as early as March 1896. Pelvimetry in its initial form was performed in 1897 by Varnier in Paris and Max Levy with L. Thumin in Berlin.[22] It was helpful to see the fetus in the uterus, but the uterine cavity without a fetus escaped visualization before they started to fill it with contrast material. This was tried only after contrast materials in the gastrointestinal tract showed that hollow spaces can be filled up without danger. The popular contrast agent at the time was bismuth so Rindfleish, in a small general hospital in Germany, introduced "a liquid paste of Bismuth" in a case showing a pathologically asymmetric uterine cavity with blockage of one of the tubes due to tubal pregnancy (1910). Soon Cary and Rubin performed hysterosalpingograms in New York, using collargol (colloidal silver) as contrast material.[23]

Visualization of the bladder, ureters, kidneys, and kidney pelves had been a longstanding desire after MacIntyre of Glasgow showed a kidney stone in July 1896.[24] Tuffier of Paris first showed the course of the ureter by introducing a metal mandrin (stylet) into it.[25] Illyés of Budapest took up the hint but added a suggestion: "It may even be better to employ a (rubber) catheter filled with Bismuth subnitrate which . . . because of the softness does not endanger the ureter during its forward movement."[26] Retrograde ureterogram and pyelogram were performed first by Voelker and Lichtenberg in Strasbourg with collargol.[27] Their method found wide acceptance, but collargol was causing irritation so Lichtenberg tried to employ oxygen as contrast in 1911.[28] In 1913 Belfield of the United States succeeded in filling the seminal vesicles with collargol through incision in the vas deferens.[29]

Since exposure times were still measured in minutes rather than seconds, the cardiovascular system was a difficult challenge because of the constant moving of the heart. Foreign bodies of metallic origin were detected in the heart, and calcium-containing plaques were visualized in arteriosclerotic vessels.[30] It would have been adventurous to inject shadow-producing material into arteries (as Haschek and Lindenthal did in Vienna), but for living creatures one had to consider embolization and toxicity.[31] Incidentally, the exposure time for Haschek's angiogram of the anatomic specimen was fifty-seven minutes.

The examination of the heart consequently remained to be pursued by fluoroscopy. The close location of the tube to the screen, however, distorted reality by magnification. To overcome this obstacle and obtain a true projection of the cardiac silhouette, the well-known cardiologist Moritz came up with the solution. He fixed the screen to standstill and moved the tube along the projection of the cardiac contour, letting only a very small central beam pass through a narrow collimator. In this way no magnification was produced and the true dimensions of the heart could either be traced on the screen with a pencil or on a paper fastened to the screen.[32] Still, the procedure was cumbersome; the suggestion of Koehler to move the tube away from the photographic plate to reduce magnification by using the more centrally located rays made sense.[33]

Observation of the motion of the heart remained for the fluoroscopist to evaluate until Sabat from the Polish city of Lwów came up with the solution, namely, to put the sequence of movements on a single plate.[34] He fastened together two parallel metallic bands to allow a slit between them. During a cardiac cycle the movement of that short segment of the heart, which was seen through the slit, could be followed. If, instead of the fluoroscopic screen, a photographic plate was put in front of the heart and pulled vertically, the final image would show a wavy curve, as the metal plates prevented exposure of the whole plate, leaving only the width of the slit exposed. The edge of the heart at that segment showed the varying states of systole, diastole, or the in-between stages of cardiac contour. Kymography was born.

There was another approach to the cardiac cycle: not from the outside, but from within to show the chambers of the heart. Chance, great ally of science, helped out occasionally. The renowned surgeon Trendelenburg reported in a medical meeting in Leipzig a case where a projectile was lodged in the heart and jumped around "as a pill shaken in a tight box," similar to what Podres in Kharkov, Russia, reported in 1898.[35] In 1907, Haecker, a young resident of the "small, flat, grey and moist" university town of Greifswald, Germany, performed experiments in dogs putting buckshot and tips of knives into the right ventricle to follow their course under fluoroscopic control as they swam through the pulmonary artery and were lodged in one of the smaller branches, or from the left ventricle down to the bifurcation of the aorta.[36] In Hamburg a year later air was introduced into guinea pigs as contrast.[37]

The most advanced trial came from Frankfurt, where Franck and Alwens injected bismuth carbonate in oil into larger veins of dogs and rabbits and watched the course of the contrast rushing through the heart.[38] They were thrilled to see the spectacle:

An impressive picture opened to the observer. . . . We will try to describe it as best we can with words. . . . The Bismuth droplets are rushing in the rabbit with great speed through the right ventricle, they circle there with fast swirling similar to a flock of mosquitoes, only to disappear through the arteria pulmonalis into the lungs . . . the larger elongated Bismuth thrombi are fragmented into smaller globules by the fast whirling in the right ventricle. . . . Observation was easier in dogs with much slower action of the heart, nevertheless, one should not forget that the Bismuth thrombi could not be seen sharply . . . as a consequence of the denser shadow of the heart.

In order to slow down the motion of the heart, they injected strophanthin to be able to see the whole cycle more accurately. "The duration of the stay of the Bismuth particles seemed to be related to their size. Those injected as a continuous thread were trapped in larger clumps for a while in the rugged inner wall. If they were taken immediately by the stream, they were circling around by chasing whirls to be then split up. The X-ray picture of the lung of the pneumothorax side is similar to a diminution of the normal lung. The summarized cross section of the vessels seems to be smaller than on the healthy side." If they injected their oil bismuth droplets into the left ventricle, the animals died within minutes, but Alwens could observe a "perfect cast of the coronaries by Bismuth" and "the X ray photograph of different organs and observation with a strong magnifying glass gives impressive sight."[39] The experience was spectacular, but inefficiency of techniques left them with a lot of imperfections: no ciné possibility was available, and in the first publication Alwens did not even try to present films; in the second one, they were hazy and unsharp.[40]

In the excitement surrounding the discovery of X rays, all kinds of schemes were published in the scientific papers to show the stomach and bowels. In animals the stomach was opened, and lead acetate was poured in through a slit; outlines of the stomach could be seen, but with predictable poor result. Another suggestion was to introduce a metallic spring into the stomach to see where it would proceed. Yet another was to let a stomach-shaped rubber bag be swallowed and then fill it with lead acetate, which would show the general shape of the stomach.[41] By the end of 1896, the first-year medical student Walter Bradford Cannon (the later leading physiologist), at the instigation of Professor Bowditch in Boston, first gave contrast-producing "buttons" to a dog, a rooster, and a frog. When he fed cats with food and Bi subnitrate, he traced for the first time the peristaltic activity and shape of parts of the stomach, including the fundus, corpus, and pylorus.[42] The next year he extended his studies in animals to watch the passing of food, vomiting, and emotional effects on peristalsis and the motion of the esophagus. All these studies would be followed throughout the next decade.[43] In 1899 Cannon helped Francis H. Williams examine human stomachs and bowels with fluoroscopy. Their findings were published in Williams's book illustrated by numerous line drawings—no photographs.[44]

At the same time in Paris, Roux and Balthasard introduced bismuth subnitrate to humans for studying the gastrointestinal tract.[45] But the first systematic study on a large scale was undertaken by Rieder in Munich.[46] He also succeeded in combining serial films in sequence into "bioroentgenography," a precursor of our ciné approach.[47]

New contrast agents were sought after toxicity was encountered with bismuth subnitrate. Ferric compounds and zirconium oxide were tried, but finally (1910) the pharmacologist Bachem in Bonn, with the clinician Guenther, found barium sulfate as the ideal contrast agent everyone was waiting.[48] Elischer in Hungary still used pure zirconium oxide, or with the admixture of air, in the stomach—our double contrast studies' predecessor.[49] The contrast he found "spread over the tumor, fills the irregularities and recesses perfectly and in this way portrays" finer details superior to the previously employed method of mixing food with bismuth subnitrate. The Swede Goesta Forsell, one of the great figures of early roentgenography, studied the gastric relief caused by the autonomous molding of the mucosal musculature (muscularis mucosae) and pointed out its independence from the movements of the stomach wall (muscularis propria).[50] Mucosal studies of the duodenum, jejunum, and colon laid the foundation for watching the finer details of the inner relief of the gastrointestinal tract.

The colon got its first examination with contrast in the retrograde fashion as we do it, with intubation of the rectum, in 1904 by Schuele in Germany.[51] The oily suspension of bismuth sulfate was soon changed to a suspension in water, giving much improved results.[52]

Although different contrast materials had their advocates, air or oxygen returned frequently as the agents not causing any toxic effects. In 1905 Robinsohn and Werndorff in Vienna injected oxygen into soft tissues to see outlines of cartilages, tendons, and tendon sheaths with good results.[53] The peritoneal cavity still presented riddles. To introduce air into the peritoneal cavity to look around with a cystoscope seemed a good idea. The shadow of the liver was separated from the diaphragm, and its outlines and those of the spleen could be identified on photographic plates. The method became so popular that it was employed for more than fifty years.[54]

Meanwhile, these diagnostic possibilities were pursued, and the physical properties of the unknown rays (cathode, Roentgen, radioactive) were clarified. Rutherford established the fact that radiation from radioactive material is by no means uniform, and he identified alpha and beta radiation in 1899. One year later Villard pointed to the third component—gamma rays. An atomic model was formulated by Rutherford in 1911. In 1912 finally the electromagnetic wave property of the X rays was identified by Laue and his associates in Germany, and the identity of the electron was recognized by J. J. Thomson in England.

At the same time there were improvements on the practical aspects of roentgenology. One was to coat both sides of the screen to support the photographic plate with fluorescent material, to add light created on the screen to the effect of X rays. This invention was so obvious that it appeared simultaneously in France, Italy, England, the United States, and Germany.[55] A motor-tilted fluoroscopy table was introduced by Caldwell in 1912. Crookes tubes underwent modification of shape and in construction of the anode. A diaphragm to cut out the nonusable disturbing radiation was recommended by one of Edison's associates.[56] Induction coils, interrupters, and static machines were employed to increase the electrical supply; then a series of coils was used (Tesla Apparatus), which enabled users to take images in ninety seconds instead of a half hour.[57] The voltages could only be estimated by the distance of the gap of the electrodes that the spark was able to jump, and the amperage was calculated by the "fatness" of the spark. The first efficient generator using alternating current (a machine similar to that which we use today) was constructed in 1907 by Snook in Philadelphia.[58]

Scattered radiation still fogged the photographs and blurred the images. To eliminate this problem in 1903, Pasche of Bern, Switzerland, recommended placing a diaphragm with a slit in the center in front of the tube and another diaphragm with a slit between the patient and the plate. If both were moved simultaneously during the exposure, the area of the travel was represented much clearer on the picture.[59] Coordination of movement of the diaphragms during the long exposure times hampered general acceptance of the device. Then came Bucky from Berlin in 1913 with a new proposal.[60] Not a single slit, but a grid formed in a honeycomb pattern was moved over the plate. The narrow metal plates of the grid were oriented toward the central ray to prevent its casting a shadow on the photograph. With movements of all kinds (straight, circular, etc.), some shadows were eliminated, yet some remained—to the chagrin of the radiologists—even though 80 percent of the scattered radiation was removed. Only by the simplification of Hollis Potter from Chicago, who employed parallel straight strips of metal instead of the honeycomb design, was the goal reached: sharp X-ray images without haziness or fogging.[61]

A little hint here, a little innovation there: everything helped. The results measured by standards known to the generation of Roentgen were spectacular. The fracture of bones did not have to be presumed; it was shown. The size of the stomach did not have to be estimated by inflating it through a rubber balloon and guessing with percussion; one could see it with the help of contrast material. Tuberculosis of the lung, still rampant, was shown on the photographic plate. But success breeds demands, and the tube still had the inherent shortcomings of being unpredictable, flickering, erratic—not uniform in performance. The outcome of each examination was always just an educated guess, accompanied by anguish as to whether it would succeed or not.

7

Technical Advances, Contrast Materials, and Radioactivity, 1913–1944

MANY TIMES progress appears from an unexpected corner, and that is exactly what made the "gas tube" obsolete. William D. Coolidge at the General Electric Company tried to find a better filament for the light bulb. Although he experimented with various metals—including copper, gold, and nickel—he finally settled on tungsten, which came to be the standard for electric lamps.[1] Of course, he also thought of using his new filament in X-ray tubes. Then he read a paper by an Austrian-born physicist named Lilienfeld, who had obtained a United States patent for a heated filament that emitted electrons even when the tube was more thoroughly evacuated of gas.

Coolidge made a shortcut in Lilienfeld's concept: if the tungsten cathode itself was heated in the X-ray tube, the whole process became simplified and more effective.[2] The penetrating power of the X rays could be controlled at will; the produced X rays were fairly homogeneous and better focused; and the X-ray photographs were both sharper and better defined. Coolidge stated that his tube differed so "radically from the tubes of the prior art . . . as to amount not so much to an improvement on prior tubes, as to an entirely new variety of tubes."[3]

Before Coolidge went public with his product, however, he offered it for clinical trial to the respected New York radiologist Lewis Gregory Cole. After a few months, Cole was so impressed with the tube that by the end of 1913 he gave a banquet in honor of the inventor. Cole described his testing of the tube, enthusiastically enumerating its advantages and declaring the Coolidge tube "undoubtedly the most important contribution to Roentgenology since the birth of the science." News traveled fast. The General Electric Company was overwhelmed with letters, telegrams, and telephone calls ordering the Coolidge tube. Customers who could not wait made the trip to the GE plant to get their specimen as soon as possible. The patent office was slow to act on Coolidge's application. It did not issue the patent until three years later.[4]

Until World War I, Belgian-made glass was the primary vehicle for X-ray images. The war sharply curtailed access to Belgium, and dangers in shipping and delays in delivery made it clear that a substitute had to be found. Cellulose nitrate was considered a solution. It had drawbacks, however. It not only curled excessively but was difficult to develop and posed a fire hazard. Nevertheless, its use continued well after the war. A major disaster at the X-ray Department of Cleveland Clinic in 1924 took 125 lives and put an end to the "play with fire." The dangerous nitrate was replaced with the safer and better cellulose acetate.[5]

According to a top expert on X-ray technology, "The development of duplitized (double coated) film, double screen and the introduction of the hot cathode tube revolutionized roentgenography."[6] Finer details were apparent in the lungs. The size and shape of the heart were clearer, and its movements were easier to follow; mucosal folds and the pathology of the esophagus, stomach, and intestines were more clearly defined. Also, a modification was added to the use of barium sulfate in the examination of the colon. In 1923, Fischer in Frankfurt introduced air on top of barium, showing pathology clearer than with the simple technique.[7]

Yet not every organ system fared well with the improved techniques. The nervous system still did not yield to the advanced X-ray technology; neither did the brain, ventricles or cysterns, entire length of the spinal cord, nor the nerves themselves. Looking for a clue, the young surgeon Dandy in Baltimore undertook the study of one hundred cases of brain tumors to find roentgenologic changes for diagnosis. To his disappointment only 6 percent of the cases were helped by radiographs, and only those that showed calcifications.[8] He considered filling the cerebral ventricles with some kind of contrast material that would produce shadow. He first experimented in dogs with a variety of solutions and suspensions— including thorium, iodide, collargol, and bismuth subnitrate—but always with fatal result. At autopsy he found edema, serosanguinal exudate, and petechial hemorrhages. Finally, wrote Dandy, "largely due to the frequent comment by Dr. Halstead [his famous chief at Johns Hopkins] on the remarkable power of intestinal gases to perforate bone that attention was drawn to its practical possibilities in the brain."[9] Dandy replaced piecemeal the cerebrospinal fluid with air and displayed films showing hydrocephalus and the degree of cortical destruction or displacement of the ventricles, or even a tumor protruding into the air-filled compartment. In 1918, Dandy proudly pronounced, "Without ventriculogram the diagnosis of hydrocephalus in children is frequently guesswork, with the ventriculogram the diagnosis is absolute." Within a year he took the additional step of showing that the ventricles could be filled through lumbar puncture; at the same time he also predicted that air could outline spinal tumors. By 1921, air myelography was successfully performed by Jacobaeus in Sweden.[10]

After Dandy's favorable experience with introduction of contrast-producing air into the ventricular system of the brain, a number of different contrast materials were explored in various organ systems. Iodine compounds appeared ever increasingly in the forefront. Of the greater researchers, the Frenchman Sicard comes preeminently to mind, yet even his achievements occurred in a rather circuitous way.

After the war Sicard returned to the Necker Hospital in Paris, where he was "*agrégé*" (assistant professor) of internal medicine and neurology. His compassion for patients' suffering was well recognized, earning him the name "the doctor of pain."[11] He was skillful with the needle in giving alcohol anesthetic injection to nerves, a talent he had developed through war-related amputations. He applied Lipiodol as an analgesic for arthritic pain and neuritis, injecting it near the nerves or into the muscles. When he observed that Lipiodol left opaque spots on X-ray photographs, he decided to "try to utilize its opacity in radiology."[12] One of his residents, Forestier, embarked on animal experiments injecting Lipiodol into muscle, skin, and peritoneal cavity. Together, Sicard and Forestier tried Lipiodol on lumbalgia and sciatica patients. The doctors watched the slow-moving substance "in hope of observing arrest of Lipiodol, the proof of an anatomic lesion for the pain."[13]

One day after examining the films they realized with horror that the Lipiodol had settled in the subarachnoid space rather than the epidural space—the needle had been pushed too far. The following two days they agonized as they waited to see whether the patient would develop meningitis. But nothing of the sort happened; in fact, the patient felt fine. They realized that instead of disaster they had hit upon a gold mine: Lipiodol could demonstrate obstructive lesions like medullary compressions. Throughout the 1920s Sicard and Forestier showed intramedullary, radicular tumors, juxtamedullary, and extramedullary tumors.[14]

And if Lipiodol was proven to be so innocuous and successful in the subarachnoid space, which cavity of the body could—or should—not be tried with the new approach? In animals they visualized the trachea and bronchi, and when they extended their studies to humans, they obtained "beautiful pictures" of the bronchial tree. They applied "supraglottic" and later "transglottic" approaches. Their films were superior to those of Chevalier Jackson, who had first tried bronchography in Philadelphia in 1919 with insufflation of bismuth powder under control of the bronchoscope.

Radiologists, and naturally French radiologists, were thrilled with the results. In the next two to three years all cavities and spaces were explored with Lipiodol as the contrast material. By 1925 there had been success with hysterosalpinogram, vesiculogram (through operative dissection of the spermatic cord; 1924), retrograde pyelogram (1925), urethrogram and localization of abscesses and sinus tracts (1922), and filling the paranasal sinuses, lacrimal ducts, and medullary cavities of bones, joints, and synovial sheaths of tendons (1923–1924). Injections into the region of the foramen ovale to help the surgeon in finding the Gasserian ganglion and injection into the pericardial sac were also performed.[15]

Sicard's and Forestier's most adventurous undertaking was injecting Lipiodol into vessels. They were encouraged by animal experiments, during which droplets passed "quite easily" through peripheral capillaries and returned through the larger veins. They saw the same quick passage in arteries of the limbs, or the renal artery; yet, after injection of Lipiodol into the common carotid artery, the animals developed respiratory syncope and died in a few minutes. In the veins Lipiodol disappeared slowly after stagnation for a while; the portal vein especially exhibited very slow flow. Lipiodol droplets were present in liver capillaries after sixty to ninety minutes. Intravascular application proved to be harmless— except for the carotid. They began human studies and showed long persistence of Lipiodol in varicose veins and also the stopping of the contrast material at the point of obstruction in the peripheral arteries of the limbs.[16]

The fervor to find suitable contrast material for various purposes inspired many researchers. In 1923 Evarts Graham, chief of surgery at Barnes Hospital in St. Louis, injected eighty-nine different compounds to visualize the gall bladder in animals, but even after two hundred experiments he and his resident Warren Cole were unable to reach their goal. Then quite unexpectedly the X ray of a certain dog injected with tetrabromo-phenolphthalein revealed the gall bladder. As Graham and Cole admired the film, it was as if— according to Cole—"we had found the traditional pot of gold at the end of the rainbow."[17] But repeated injection of the same material did not yield the same good result. They reviewed the protocol but could observe no difference in administration of the drug. The animal caretaker was asked whether the star dog had been treated in any special way, but he denied it. After pressure from Cole, the caretaker admitted that he had forgotten to feed the particular animal on the morning of the injection. This gave the clue: in all other animals food resulted in the contraction of the gall bladder with the resulting emptying of the collected contrast material; with no food, the contrast stayed in the gall bladder.

These experiments led finally to showing what had so long escaped visualization.[18] A few years later the substitution of bromide with iodide in the molecule was accepted as the material of choice.

Also in 1923, physicians at the Mayo Clinic came upon an easy solution to the riddle of demonstrating the urinary collecting system, bypassing the cumbersome method of retrograde studies with its inherent danger of infection or irritation. They began studies on an active outpatient department for syphilis, which they treated with large doses of 10 percent NaI (50–250 ml). One of the team—Rowntree—had had previous but unsuccessful experiences with iodoform emulsion in oil tried for bronchography. Utilizing the excellent contrast property of iodine, he recommended that films be taken of syphilitic patients after the injection of NaI.[19] Since it was known that the compound was excreted with the urine, the team could thus have clinical trials without resorting to time-consuming animal experiments.[20] Rowntree's recommendation bore results, and intravenous pyelography was born.

When the Mayo team followed the injection with fluoroscopy, they noted that "the cephalic vein has the appearance of a steel wire, from the point of injection of the iodide at the elbow to the juncture of the cephalic vein with the subclavian. . . . In all probability with variations in the technique important results will be obtained with regard to the venous return and the peripheral arterial circulation. In the study of aneurysm and of arterio-venous anastomosis it should also be of value." They failed to follow their own advice, however.

It was probably not these lines, but rather discussions with Walter Alwens in Frankfurt (chapter 6) that encouraged Berberich and Hirsch to embark on experiments for visualizing vessels.[21] The search for contrast material was still the first step to take. Calcium compounds, sodium, and strontium salts of halogens were tried in rabbits. Water-soluble strontium bromide became their choice. Berberich and Hirsch successfully demonstrated the basilar vein as well as the first human arteriogram with water-soluble material. The radial artery with its small division was demonstrated, but severe pain and occasional infiltrates discouraged the researchers, and their altered professional circumstances broke up the promising beginning.[22]

Rowntree's presentation on intravenous pyelography and the ensuing comment most likely inspired Barney Brooks, hailed as the

"Essential Teacher of Surgery" at Barnes Hospital, where Graham and Cole conducted their experiments. Brooks's injections of 10 ml of 100 percent NaI solution into the femoral artery with surgical cut-down of patients with gangrene of the leg obtained nice angiograms.[23] Despite favorable comments by his colleagues, Brooks claimed that his thermocouple method of demonstrating blockage of arteries was "absolutely harmless and I am convinced that the more it is used. . . the less often it will be necessary to resort to injection of the arteries. . . . I do not believe that the method is a safe one to be indiscriminately used."[24]

Although not often in science do many things occur at the same time, the year 1923 was exceptional. The return to civilian pursuits after World War I let energies of productive minds burst. In one single year medicine saw the solution of myelography, bronchography, salpingography, cholecystography, and intravenous pyelography. With timid advances and some disappointments, some progress was made in arteriography. The real push came from Egas Moniz, who had attended medical school in Lisbon and then spent some years in France studying neurology with Sicard. Moniz settled in his native Portugal, where he combined a chair in neurology in Lisbon with a successful political career. He served as a representative of his native district, ambassador to Spain, foreign minister, and leader of the Portuguese delegation to the Versailles peace treaty negotiations. After a clash with an important politician, he returned to his chair of neurology. But a born leader cannot rest idle. Moniz's "desire to obtain new facts, something useful and still not known," became an obsession. His goal was to prove that large oral doses of bromides might show up in the brain. When his efforts failed, he thought of showing pathology with visualization of the vascular architecture or its distortion in the brain, by injecting bromide compounds into the arteries. First in meticulous experiments with dogs and then with anatomical specimens of human brains, he became acquainted with the blood supply in normal and pathological conditions. He borrowed severed heads from the anatomical institute (which lacked X-ray facilities) and brought them to his institute, injecting the arteries with contrast, taking the films, and making the gruesome return trip in a taxicab to the anatomical institute.[25]

In human trials, he soon exchanged bromides with an atomic weight of only 80 for iodides with an atomic weight of 127, which gave much better contrast. Also, bromides applied arterially caused headaches and fever, which iodides did not. Finally, in mid-1927, using iodides, Moniz demonstrated the Sylvian group of arteries and the carotid siphon. Great showman that Moniz was, he departed the next week to Paris to present his films to members of the Neurological Society. There he encountered his old teacher Sicard. Surrounded by students and with the self-consciousness of his past years' successes, Sicard said: "Oh you are here Monsieur Moniz. Is there something you bring to us from Portugal to localize brain tumors?" Sicard became less sarcastic when Moniz showed him the films in the line of research he had failed. Moniz was greeted with resounding acclaim.[26]

Moniz and his close associate Alemida Lima had injected 5 ml of 22% NaI through surgical cut-down into both carotid arteries and had taken two to three lateral projections of the skull. Their machinery was not sufficient to yield short enough exposures for anterio-posterior projection. Moniz published a monograph with ninety cases of cerebral angiograms, some followed clinically and some through surgery or autopsy. Babinski, the world-known master of neurology, supplied the congratulatory preface, and Moniz became a celebrity in neurology and radiology.[27]

After a 1928 meeting in Lisbon at which Moniz demonstrated his cases, the urologist Raynaldo dos Santos asked whether the method could be tried in the extremities. "But certainly," answered Moniz, "and with the least of apprehension. I think it would be a credit to your account."[28] Dos Santos jumped at the project and performed arteriographies in a wide variety of diagnoses: arteriosclerosis, aneurysms, osteomyelitis due to tuberculosis, and syphilis. After a long series of cases he embarked on the bold adventure of piercing the lumbar aorta from the back with a long needle. When he filled the abdominal aorta with contrast material, even some of its branches became visible.[29] In 1931 Dos Santos and then Moniz employed radioactive Thorotrast for arteriography (but not for aortography) because of its excellent contrast and absence of pain and because they believed that Thorotrast did not cause any harm, which later proved false. Even the minimal radioactivity had its bad consequences. Nevertheless, Dos Santos and Moniz made remarkable strides in the development of arteriography and aortography.

The world still did not catch up, however. Critics talked about the dangers and questioned the usefulness of the method. To speak about dangers was not unrealistic, since the risk of the needle-sticking of the aorta and the finding of an innocuous contrast material that would deliver good pictures were still unresolved. Caution when employing a high concentration of NaI or Thorotrast was well justified. And then came the turning point. The American Swick, working in Berlin with Binz and von Lichtenberg, came up with the practically harmless organic iodine compound, uroselectan, for urography. Uroselectan had obvious implications for angiography as well.[30]

Swick's report happened to be published in the same issue of a medical journal as one by Forssmann about experiments with catheterization of the heart.[31] As a medical student in Berlin, Forssmann had been humiliated when, during a class on percussion as a diagnostic tool, he was unable to properly locate the heart of a patient with dextrocardia.[32] He reasoned that if he could inject contrast material into the heart, he could reach a better understanding of its real dimensions and workings. As a young intern in the small hospital's emergency room, he made a cut-down of his own antecubital vein (nobody wanted to participate in that experiment), introduced a ureter catheter, pushed it way into the right atrium, walked up a flight of stairs to the X-ray department, and took the first film demonstrating a catheter in the human heart.

With some trepidation, he tried to inject contrast material through the catheter. He knew that if anything should go wrong with the catheter he could pull it out, but once the contrast material touched the endocardium, no one could predict what would happen.[33] No ill effect was sensed, but nothing showed up on the film either— obviously he had introduced too small an amount and the contrast had become diluted.

With experiments in dogs, however, he succeeded in demonstrating the first right ventricular angiogram through catheter introduction. His otherwise talented chief, Sauerbruch, at the time took Forssmann's approach as a gimmick. After a sharp encounter—both were headstrong—he ousted the younger man as a fraud. Another strike of bad luck occurred at a medical meeting when Forssmann demonstrated his catheter-introduced films. His films showing the right ventricle of animals, reaching as far as the pulmonary arteries, had to follow the presentation of the well-respected professor Janker.[34] After Janker's cine films of needle-introduced contrast material into the left ventricle of rabbits, what chance had the young resident against the well-known professor? Also, catheterization of the heart was thought to lack any useful purpose. Some mentioned ethical considerations, others accused him of "lack of conscience," while others just laughed.[35]

Trying to catch the fleeting second of motion was not quite new in the 1930s; it was an ongoing effort. As early as 1897, just one year after Roentgen's discovery and about the time of the beginning of motion pictures made for entertainment, the Scotsman MacIntyre from Glasgow took photographic images from the screen in sequence with an ordinary camera. Another rapid-sequence approach had been tried in 1914 by Lewis Gregory Cole in New York, who had employed a long roll of film coupled with a semiautomatic mechanism advancing the film at the pressing of a lever. Fifty films could be made in rapid succession and, if projected one after another, they suggested the motion of the organ. Cineroentgenography, as we know it, had two industrious proponents in the 1930s: Janker in Germany and Reynolds in England. Each conducted good clinical work, but the shortcoming of their machinery made it impossible for them to both watch the object and take the films. Image amplifiers were nonexistent as yet. Reynolds succeeded in getting sixty frames per second, which he could run for sixteen seconds in his cardiac patients. He theorized that with a slow-motion film he could better analyze the heart's action.[36]

Even if cinematography resolved certain problems with moving organs, there was a remaining riddle. How could the disturbing shadows overlying the object of interest be eliminated? In 1914 the Polish radiologist Karol Mayer tried to smear the shadows of the ribs by moving the tube while the film was exposed in order to have a clearer outline of the heart. One year later the Italian Baese's objective was to localize battle-inflicted bullets in the body by moving the tube and film in opposite directions during exposure.

In 1921 the Frenchman Bocage applied for a patent with a similar arrangement, but with more precise execution. Although Bocage's idea was sound, he did not succeed in building his machine for another seventeen years. A few months after his description the same idea was patented by two other Frenchmen, Portes and Chausse. The American Kieffer applied for a patent in 1929 on his machine, but the stock market crash and ill health prevented him from pursuing his goal for another six years.[37] Vallebona in Genoa rotated the skull rather than the tube and films, although later he changed the arrangement with head fixed, tube and film moving.[38] The radiologist Ziedses des Plantes of Utrecht, Holland, aimed for the same goal, although Grossmann from Berlin came up with the simplest and most practical solution of tomography and set up the equipment with the help of the clinician Chaoul in 1935.[39] Lung cavities, abscesses, and bone pathology were at last neatly defined and specified.

Another innovation was worked out by Ziedses des Plantes. The problem was the same as with tomography: how to eliminate overlying shadows. Stereoscopy was one of the answers, and a similar solution was the "plastic" or "relief-type" images produced in 1906 by the Hungarian Bela Alexander by making a direct copy of a glass-plate photograph and superimposing another taken from a slightly different angle. The product was a photograph suggesting a three-dimensional image.[40] Des Plantes started from the fact that if you take a film, make a positive copy, then superimpose one upon the other, the blacks of one will blank out the whites of the other—and make the copy of them neutral—and thus, the original image will be wiped out. But if something shows on the second film that was not present when the first film was taken, then it will be seen on the copy—without the rest of the shadows. In short, the newly introduced object would be represented clearly.[41] In angiography the method proved to be excellent: one could see the contrast-filled vessels without the overlying bones.

Visualization of the cardiac ventricles still had not been achieved. It waited for the Cuban Augustin Castellanos, who realized in 1937 that in infants congenital heart disease could be diagnosed by injecting contrast material.[42] One year later the Americans Robb and Steinberg made a series of films in Boston with angiograms showing the cardiac ventricles. But how difficult it was! They lacked cassette changers, and serial sequences could not be achieved. So they first determined the circulation time, injected contrast material into both antecubital veins, waited for an agonizing twenty or less seconds, and then snapped a single film. They were not always successful, yet in 80 percent of the cases they came up with creditable images: both ventricles, even the ascending aorta, were well visualized.[43] After having shown 215 angiocardiograms without fatality, Robb and Steinberg presented their findings to the American Roentgen Ray Society in Atlantic City in 1938. Many of the attending doctors hardly believed their ears and eyes. Dr. Steinberg's wife, sitting in the audience as a spectator, overheard the remark at the beginning of their talk: "This is not true. They are lying."[44]

These were great advances. The cardiac ventricles inside, which both Leonardo da Vinci and Forssmann dreamed about, finally were visualized. But not the valves. The lungs were well demonstrated it seemed, but not the infarcts or many times the emphysematous blebs. The stomach, duodenum, and colon were clearly examined with spot films, but frequently the source of the bleeding could not be pinpointed. It was great to see the gallbladder and gallstones, but the liver? True, the liver and spleen were demonstrated as they collected thorium in their reticuloendothelial cells—but only in animal experiments.[45] The doctors would not have been happy to irradiate their patients by the gamma rays of thorium. The kidneys and the urinary collecting system were fairly well demonstrated, but renal hypertension was unexplained.

As for the central nervous system? The ventricles were visualized, but patients had to be strapped into a ferocious-looking giant ring-like structure that could turn them upside down to collect the air into the desired corner of the posterior horn. The brain itself was the supreme challenge. Nothing could be identified, not even the white or grey matter, to say nothing of the cerebral nuclei. Bones were well demonstrated, but not the muscles and tendons. Much had been revealed by the 1930s, but much was still unknown.

But from what sciences could clarification be expected? Physicists paid increasing interest to the evermore mystifying secrets of the atoms, especially the discovery that they were not indivisible entities. In the first two decades of the century a select group of physicists came closer to unraveling the questions of composition of matter, and step by step they identified the electrons (Thomson in 1897), the alpha rays (Rutherford in 1899), and the gamma rays (Villard in 1900). In 1913 the atom was finally recognized as a miniature solar system by the Dane Niels Bohr. Whether atoms would play any role in diagnostic medicine nobody could predict, but the fact that gamma rays were akin to X rays pointed to possible analogies. The solutions offered by physicists seemed only to complicate matters. Rutherford, the most active of all the scientists, found something surprising almost every month. When one of his envious colleagues remarked, "You are lucky, Rutherford, you always ride at the crest of the waves," Rutherford retorted, "Yes, but I am the one who makes the waves."

So it must have been a great challenge and honor for the Budapest chemist von Hevesy to work in Rutherford's laboratory. As Hevesy was known to have followed chemical properties of lead, adding radium D to it and having traced its radioactivity, Rutherford assigned him the task of separating lead from its isotope radium D. Hevesy was unable to do so; all experiments showed the same reactions for both. Only at one point were they different: radium D was radioactive, whereas lead was not. Consequently, with minute amounts of radium D in the mixture with lead, the compound could be checked with an electroscope on account of its radioactivity. Lead could be followed wherever it went.[46] Hevesy watered plants with lead solution with added traces of radium D and followed their distribution by checking their course with an electroscope.[47] That was the first tracer study in a living organism. Later, Hevesy turned to studies with rabbits; he injected radium E, which being "Bismuthotrop" mixed well with bismuth, important in those days in the therapy of syphilis. He thus followed the accumulation and elimination of bismuth, measuring the radioactivity of its accompanying RaE: the first animal tracer study.[48] Most likely it was at that time that Hevesy became suspicious that his landlady was serving the remainder of the same dish day after day, so he sprinkled the food with a little thorium B and checked the radioactivity on the next occasion with his electroscope. The landlady noticed it, and Hevesy had to leave.[49]

One year later, in 1927, the Boston cardiologist Blumgart checked circulation time by injecting RaC into patients and measuring the radioactivity of blood samples with a small ionizing chamber.[50] In the February 1934 issue of *Nature,* an article by Frédéderic Joliot and Irène Curie announced: "Our latest experiments have shown a very striking fact: when an aluminum foil is irradiated, the emission of positrons (from a Polonium source) does not cease immediately. . . . The foil remains radioactive. . . . We observed the same phenomenon with Boron and Magnesium. . . . The Transmutation has given birth to new radio elements emitting positrons."[51] In Rome, Fermi read the paper and set to work immediately. By May, only three months later, he published the results of his own experiments with artificial radioactive elements by bombardment of pure elements with neutrons obtained from a source of radon.[52] Years later Fermi, Joliot, and Curie received the Nobel Prize for their creation of new radioactive elements.

Using Fermi's ^{32}P as a tracer, Hevesy in 1935 fed rats radioactive ^{32}P and concluded that "the formation of bones is a dynamic process, involving continuous loss and replacement."[53] (At that time, atomic weights were expressed after the chemical sign, as P^{32}, but they are standardized here according to the current form.) Hevesy's experiments proved that the "tracer" concept carried great value and probably could be extended to other areas. Hevesy extended his experiences. He tagged red blood cells with ^{32}P and then injected a sample into other animals. A few minutes later the dilution of the radioactive element in the recipient animal indicated the blood volume. The method was eventually applied to humans too.[54] The turnover rate of nucleic acid was followed with the tracer method as ^{32}P was incorporated into DNA, and the turnover rate of dental enamel was also observed.[55] In November 1936 a scientific meeting took up the proposal "What Physics Can Do for Biology and Medicine."[56]

In Berkeley, California, next to the famous cyclotron, the very young neurologist Hamilton, well versed in studies with radioactive elements, reached his heart's desire: experiments with the human thyroid. With a fairly pure ^{131}I source from Lawrence's cyclotron, it became evident that the accumulation of ingested radioactive iodine in the thyroid gland depended on the working conditions of the gland, pointing to its function. Thus, the "uptake" also gained clinical diagnostic significance.[57] It was hoped that ^{131}I would seek out and show the location of metastases of thyroid carcinoma, but that hope proved to be valid in only 25 percent of the cases. Medical application of radioactive isotopes gained momentum, but certain events alien to medical thinking blocked further development in this line.

A change in attitudes was initiated by the famous letter of Einstein to President Franklin D. Roosevelt in August 1939. Einstein called attention to the possibility of a nuclear chain reaction in uranium and pointed out that "a single bomb of this type carried by boat and exploded in a port, might very well destroy the whole port together with some of the surrounding territories."[58] After seven months with no promise of monetary support, Einstein wrote a second letter in March 1940: "Since the outbreak of war, interest in Uranium has intensified in Germany. I have now learned that research there is being carried out in great secrecy." When the United States entered the war in December 1941, the atomic sciences were drawn increasingly into the center of attention. Because of the strategic significance of knowledge in the field, a lid was put upon most scientific publications or research with radioisotopes in medical matters, in order to keep the Axis uninformed. The Berkeley cyclotron, which once produced radioactive isotopes for medical use, was used instead to make plutonium.

Much of Europe and the Far East was already in shambles. The nations put all their energy into the fatal struggle. Everything was touched by the war atmosphere. Scientific imagination, abstract reasoning, and experimental activity were all drained into the war effort.

8

More Technology Helps to See More: 1940s, 1950s, and 1960s

IN THE 1930s, the well-developed nations of the world contributed to the advancement of the sciences. By the following decade, most of the world was engaged in war. Medical personnel was called for military service; scarce supplies could not be spared for experimental animals. Many scientists were persecuted or perished in the turmoil. Quiet concentration and laboratory work were far-gone dreams in the war-torn countries.

North America, although affected by the war, did not suffer invasion or actual combat. Consequently, scientific activity in those fateful years—and even in the postwar years—was concentrated in the United States and Canada. Advancement in physics, chemistry, and medicine was accomplished to a large extent there.

Several innovations in X-ray technology were introduced during the war. In 1942 Russell H. Morgan from Chicago announced his solution for timing the exposure of films automatically, terminating the delivery of radiation after the proper quantity had been delivered.[1] Both the use of the phototimer and the automatic processing of films introduced by the Pako Corporation in 1942 (and subsequent refinements of Kodak X-omat in 1956) facilitated work in X-ray departments considerably.[2] The real big leap forward, however, came with the image amplifier and television. Coltman of the Westinghouse Company described a new vacuum tube in 1948 capable of intensifying the original image; in 1952 such a device was put on the market with a gain of 200 times in brightness. In years the performance of image amplifiers achieved 4-, 5-, and even 6,000 gain.

A competition for image amplifiers came with television. The idea of televised transmission of pictures was conceived as early as 1908 by Campbell Swinton of Scotland, who described his thoughts in an address to the London Roentgen Society in 1911. Experiments were undertaken in this line by Baird in England and Jenkins in the United States in 1923. In the same year a Russian immigrant, Vladimir Zworykin, working with the RCA laboratories in the United States, constructed his "iconoscope camera tube," which became so indispensable for electronic television transmission. Electric and Musical Industries (EMI) in Great Britain set up a research group for television and could boast of the first public service in London in 1936. In the United States public television broadcasting started in 1941. It was soon realized that TV could be used for intensification of X-ray images.

Russell Morgan, by then at Johns Hopkins Medical School in Baltimore, coupled TV equipment with the screen in 1948, and one year later Richard Chamberlain and Sam Seal, working with the engineers of RCA Victor, coupled a newly developed tube with the screen and embarked on ciné recordings with hitherto unseen distinction. The brightness could hit a mark of 50,000 gain.[3] In the same year Janker in Bonn achieved image amplification employing TV. Surgical instructors at the Medical Center of the University of Kansas employed TV in the 1950s. Bronchoscopy was shown on TV by Soulas in Paris in 1956, and the retina soon could be shown on the TV screen.

Spot filming had been used in the late 1930s but was hampered by inaccurate exposures that rendered films either underexposed or overexposed. Phototiming put an end to this. Shockproofing of dangerous high-voltage lines, introduction of sophisticated tables that could be tilted from vertical to horizontal positions with ease, and the use of valve tube rectifiers all had a favorable impact on radiology. It is difficult to imagine today what a difference those improvements meant. One could walk around the X-ray rooms safely without danger of electrical execution from high-voltage cables; one could throw away the red goggles that were once required to keep the adaptation sensitive (but made the radiologist look like a space alien). One could walk into the fluoroscopy room without wasting half an hour to acquire the appropriate degree of adaptation. One could rely on spot films for examination of the GI tract; and one could record coughing, swallowing, and cardiac revolutions on ciné films for play and replay at later times and could slow the movements for study. The details seen with image amplification on the TV were immeasurably brighter than with previous machinery.

When dates are given for the introduction of new technology, they represent the year of introduction, probably with only a single prototype or experimental model. Mass production and distribution of successful final models could take five to ten years before an invention reached general utilization. The innovations of the 1940s consequently became well accepted only by the 1950s and sometimes even the 1960s. The fact remains that a new era opened for radiology and lifted the specialty to a higher level of performance, just at a time that advances in medicine and especially in surgery made the medical profession more demanding for more accurate diagnosis. The recently developed heart surgery in particular leaned heavily on roentgenologic diagnosis, which derived mainly from cardiac catheterization and angiography.

Back in the early 1930s Forssmann, surrounded in Germany with criticism and deafening silence, was pushed aside from further research as an academic outcast, but his cardiac catheterization efforts found new champions in Prague, Lisbon, Brazil, Cuba, and Paris. Yet when Amheuille and his group presented their films of pulmonary angiograms in 1935, the leading French cardiologists piled argument upon argument against the procedure, despite the fact that no mishap was encountered in one hundred cases.[4] Encouraged by Amheuille's report, two residents at Columbia University in New York embarked on a project to examine systematically the cardiopulmonary function in normal and sick persons. Cournand (a student of Amheuille's), together with Dickinson Richards, conducted measurements of cardiac output, blood volume, intraventricular and intra-atrial pressure, respiratory gas exchange, blood gases, and pH. Meanwhile, they not only improved the cardiac catheter but even designed a double-lumen catheter to measure pressures simultaneously in the atrium and ventricle. Between 1940 and 1944, they examined 103 individuals without a single unpleasant experience. They proceeded in their studies with great caution. Only after becoming familiar with atrial exploration, they advanced their catheter into the right ventricle; two more years elapsed before they stretched it into the pulmonary artery.[5] With their meticulous technique and circumspect evaluations of the mass of data, they opened a new chapter in cardiopulmonary physiology and pathology. Following their lead, McMichael and Sharpey-Schafer in England examined patients in circulatory shock, successfully studying vasovagal reflex and cardiac failure in 353 catheterizations; yet the gurus of cardiology shook their heads over the method.[6] Despite such misgivings, pressure-readings and angiography were practiced eventually in advanced centers, and the whole venous system and the right heart were explored—but the arterial system remained reluctant to reveal its details.

To inject arteries of the extremities and the carotids was accepted procedure in university hospitals; but visceral arteries, the ascending aorta, and the arch and the left ventricle were not ready for angiography. Trials and modes of approach were numerous, but none yielded the expected results. To reach the ramifications of the aorta, catheters were introduced through surgical cut-down of the femoral artery by Fariñas in Cuba in 1940 and by Radner in Sweden in 1948.[7] In 1951 Peirce in the United States inserted a polyethylene tube through a wide trocar into the femoral artery, but the tube was nonopaque and rigid, unsatisfactory for practical purposes.[8]

More daring approaches were deflated before they could take off on a larger scale. In Germany, Euler's 1949 attempted periesophageal puncture of the aorta was less than popular.[9] The direct percutaneous puncture of the left ventricle or ascending aorta by the Cubans Ponsdomenech and Beato-Nuñez in 1951 could not gain general acceptance despite their fifty-six cases without mishap.[10] In 1950 both retrograde catheterization of the left ventricle by Zimmermann and Limon and the left ventricular intracavitary ECG tracings of the Mexican Sodi-Pallares represented trials that few followed.[11] All represented tentative probings into the yet-unexplored arterial side of the circulation, but no safe, easy-to-employ methodology emerged from them.

The 1949 approach used by Joensson (Jönsson) of Sweden was probably the most original of the attempts made to reach the aortic arch and its branches. He introduced double-coaxial needles into the common carotid artery retrograde, facing the aorta. He then withdrew the inner narrower needle and replaced it with a fine silver thread. With its guidance, he pushed the needle over the thread gently into the aorta, then withdrew the thread, and at last he could inject contrast material to visualize the arch and its branches.[12] Visualization of both the aortic arch and thoracic aorta was accomplished, but the vascular supply of the organs was still amiss. That was the state of affairs in the late 1940s, when a solution came from Sweden, the lucky corner of Europe untouched by the devastations of war.

The question of how to introduce a catheter into the arterial system was put before one of the conferences in the X-ray department of the respected Karolinska Institut in Stockholm. One of the residents, Ivar Seldinger, suggested the following method: Introduce a needle through a side hole of a catheter into the artery, withdraw the needle, introduce a wire from the outside end of the catheter, forward it into the desired point, withdraw the wire after the catheter was pushed forward, and thus reach the goal. But the side hole carried the risk of rupture. Also, the contrast material became diluted because it reached the end hole as well as the side hole. In Seldinger's own words: "Once after an unsuccessful attempt of using that technique, I stood in the lab quite sad with the three items in my hand: the needle, the guide wire, and the catheter; and suddenly I was aware of how they should be properly used."[13] The solution was really quite simple. A needle was introduced into the artery, then a guide wire slipped into the needle from the distal end of it; the needle was then withdrawn and a catheter threaded over the wire into the artery; when the wire was finally pulled, the catheter was in place.[14] The method was easy to follow, no cut-down was necessary, and the catheter could be pushed as far as needed from the usual femoral artery approach. Seldinger and soon

Oedman (also from Stockholm) started to map out the arterial tree; others followed in rapid sequence. Within a few years the vascular organs could be visualized in their finest ramifications, including the coronary arteries.[15]

The 1956 Nobel Prize for Cournand, Richards, and Forssmann marked the recognition of the scientific world for major achievements in visualization of the organs of the human body.[16] It was also the time when people started to ponder the menace—or possible benefit—of nuclear power. The surprising Hungarian revolt against totalitarian rule raised the question of who are going to be the leaders in possession of an almost unlimited potential of destruction and benefit. The power of the bombs blasted in 1945 at Hiroshima and Nagasaki and the experiments at the Bikini Atoll in 1954 were shocking, yet newspaper articles and TV reports predicted that such forces might be harnessed for medicine. Perhaps those mysterious powers might even extend lives through the understanding of nuclear construction.

Scant reports and fuzzy speculations prevailed about the medical use of radioactive isotopes until August 1946, when the Atomic Energy Act "released isotopes from military control."[17] A deluge of articles about radioactivity ensued: between 1946 and 1951, there were a total of 3,200, of which 949 discussed medical possibilities.[18] Once attention was drawn to the available radioactive isotopes ^{32}P and ^{131}I in regard to thyroid problems, bone pathology, or leukemia, they became cherished targets for research. Difficulties hampered efforts, however. The only available measuring device—the Geiger-Mueller counter—was not sufficiently sensitive, with less than 1 percent efficiency for gamma ray detection.[19] Also, recording data was a slow and laborious process as the probe was moved from point to point, handheld in front of the thyroid gland. Then came reports in 1947 from Germany that H. Kallman had achieved increased sensitivity with a block of naphthalene, the bug-repellent luminescent material, in front of a photomultiplier tube.[20] Gamma rays or any charged particle caused scintillations (light flashes) in naphthalene, and these, picked up with the photomultiplier, could be measured, along with the energy level of the emitted gamma rays. This device converted the subjective method of observing scintillations on a screen with the naked eye to a measurable dimension. By 1949 Robert Hofstadter at General Electric laboratories had discovered that if naphthalene was replaced with a thallium-activated NaI crystal, sensitivity was further increased; with later modifications he improved on the Geiger-Mueller counter ninety-five times.[21] Upon Cassen's suggestion, researchers at the University of California at Los Angeles devised a free-floating arm, coupled with a scintillation counter, which when driven slowly over the neck of the horizontally lying patient, could pick up the activity of the thyroid gland; the addition of a moving pen could provide a map for the endocrinologist, as well as give information about the relative radioiodine contents of accumulation in the gland. The prototype of this design, ready in 1951, opened a new chapter in nuclear medicine.[22] The study of radioactivity thus stepped over from tracer techniques and laboratories into practical imaging of organs.

The problem with the rectilinear scanner was its slow performance. Anger, in the Donner Laboratory of Medical Physics, worked on the idea of somehow constructing a device that would eliminate the moving arm and take pictures from a stable source, similar to a photographic camera. Anger finally achieved his goal in 1958, and in 1964 a twelve-inch camera was announced to the public with much-improved efficiency.[23] Industry was slow to become interested in Anger's invention but eventually made further improvements that led to a decrease in patient dosage and to the use of low-energy gamma-emitting ^{134}I and ^{99m}Tc.[24] Radioactive technetium was introduced in 1964 by Harper, a desirable radioactive element with low-gamma energy level and no beta emission. Also, its half life of six hours ensured rapid decline of radiation in the patient's body. All kinds of radioactive elements were tried for imaging of different organs, but after elimination of several impractical materials, it was found that ^{99m}Tc coupled with certain compounds could seek out desired organs. Technetium diphosphonate became the imaging material for bones; sulfur colloid for liver and spleen; macroaggregates for lung; and pertechnetate for brain, thyroid, and kidney. Of course, advances continue as better materials are tested. How long ^{57}Ga, ^{201}Tl, or others will stay with us—before being replaced with better elements—will depend on future investigations.

Nuclear imaging studies opened up a wide array of diagnostic possibilities. Tumors or infection of bones not seen in X-ray films were suddenly recognized. Liver and spleen at long last showed metastases, infarcts, and traumatic rupture. Lung scans revealed to our surprise how much had been missed with chest X rays in cases of emphysema, infarct, and tumor. Kidney pathology, sometimes not recognized, was demonstrated, as were brain tumors and infarcts never perceived before. One other thrilling aspect of research with radioactive material was its power to reveal metabolic and chemical changes in the organs and cells. The first in this line of inquiry was the thyroid gland, and its function, to be followed by investigations of the liver and the kidneys. Doctors could detect disease even before microscopic changes had occurred. As Henry Wagner pointed out: "Nuclear medicine is teaching us that structure and function are but two aspects of a unitary process."[25] Sophisticated machinery made it possible even to pursue dynamic studies, pointing to malfunctioning of the myocardium and showing the location of infarcts or scars.

No matter how rewarding those avenues might have been, radioactive isotopes as well as X rays had two major drawbacks. First of all, both delivered harmful radiation, which caused fear in the general public, leading to ever-increasing publicity in the news media, and erupting occasionally in angry demonstrations. Although the medical sciences moved into broader applications of the recently experienced advances, yet it would have been helpful to eliminate the radiation hazard. The second drawback of nuclear medicine and roentgenology was that they rendered only black and white silhouettes of organs. Color, so important for diagnosis, escaped observation.

Photography had enjoyed color since the early 1930s. Eastman in Rochester showed the first color motion picture in 1928, and Bell Laboratories started to experiment with color TV in 1929. First to work with color in X-ray photography was an Irishman, Donovan, who expressed his thinking to the Cork Clinical Society in 1950, reminding the audience that his color "tagging" of films was similar to staining in microscopic techniques—in other words, the colors did not represent the natural color of organs, but rather an arbitrary color depending on absorption of the Roentgen rays.[26] An

American group from Louisville, Kentucky, soon followed; it was their opinion that instruction of students could be greatly enhanced with color. In the same year of 1951, French, German, and Japanese researchers followed suit. Bonnan of California described further improvements, yet even he admitted that for seasoned radiologists color might not represent a great advantage.[27]

To look at natural color in the inside of tubes or cavities was to resort to endoscopy. With appropriate instruments one could see hyperemia, blood, pallor, jaundice, and scars. The difficulty was that all those instruments consisted of rigid metal tubes. One could look into the pharynx, larynx, urinary bladder, or rectum, but when it was necessary to view longer and tortuous structures like the esophagus, sigmoid, or smaller ramifications of the bronchial tree, something longer and more flexible was called for. Schindler of Berlin enlisted the assistance of the instrument maker Wolff, who set to work on a flexible gastroscope. Together they developed a tube that was half rigid metal and half flexible rubber. The whole length contained more than forty lenses, which bounced the image from the stomach to the observer's eyes. They showed their sixth and final prototype to a medical society meeting in Munich in 1932.[28]

Although the success of the partly flexible gastroscope was undeniable, the only beneficiary was the stomach. The sigmoid and the trachea were still examined with short rigid scopes—as far as they could be pushed without danger. A Dutchman, an Englishman, and a Pakistani set change in motion. Van Heel described the transmission of light through glass fibers coated with lacquer along a curved path.[29] Incidentally, transmission of light through a curved stream of water was known to Tyndall in England in 1870, and the whole concept of transmitting light through a curved surface of glass had been patented in England as early as 1923 by Baird, one of the originators of television transmission.[30] Hopkins in London added the suggestion in 1954 that "very fine glass fibers should also possess this property and have the added advantage of flexibility."[31] In their experiments Hopkins and the Pakistani Kapany realized that 0.001-inch-diameter fibers transmitted light with small loss.

Coming from South Africa, Hirschowitz was working with rigid gastroscopes and sigmoidoscopes in Ann Arbor as a resident. When he read the articles of Van Heel and Hopkins, he remarked that those papers had "struck a spark."[32] Together with Curtiss and Peters he produced glass fibers of microscopic width in a one-meter-long bundle. His fibers could transmit only fuzzy images, however, because light was lost to the neighboring fibers. Under the microscope the lacquer coating of Van Heel showed irregularities and the images were scrambled and dim. When Curtiss came up with the idea of replacing the lacquer with a coat of glass with lesser refractory power, "all the wise men in the physics basement lunch group laughed at him."[33] But they did not give up.

After much patient experimentation the goal was reached: two hundred thousand frail fibers were properly coated, each one measuring a mere fifteen microns in diameter, with a light loss of only 0.00004.[34] They were bunched into a flexible bundle of about a finger's breadth (consider that the hair on our head counts not more than one hundred thousand threads), and they could bounce light and image with clarity, color, and good resolution. To prove the point, Hirschowitz showed President Lincoln's picture on a small stamp through the fiberscope with clear-cut details to the audience of the American Gastroenterology Society meeting in May 1957.[35] The presentation was a success, yet the industry was hesitant. It took another three years before manufacturing for commercial use began.

The Japanese approached the problem from another angle. They constructed a tiny camera that could be forwarded into the stomach for pictures of the gastric mucosa: the gastrocamera was introduced by Uji and the Japanese Olympus Optical Corporation in 1950.[36] The disadvantage was that the camera could not be aimed: pictures were not centered, and the operator could not be certain of capturing points of highest interest. Also, the images were only 0.5 cm in diameter, smaller than desirable for casual inspection.

Fiberoptics, on the other hand, were thriving. Hirschowitz had gained tremendous impact over the original goal of Schindler. With further technical improvements, the entire length of the colon and the duodenum could be visualized by direct inspection, thus opening the possibility of cannulating the papilla of Vater with endoscopic retrograde choledocho-pancreatography (ERCP), removal of polyps in the colon, and somewhat later diagnosis of such elusive conditions as angiodysplasia.[37] Visualization of the bronchial tree to considerable depth was achieved all the way out to the finer ramifications of the bronchi, never reached previously. Biopsy, electrocautery, and Argon-laser transmission through the fibers were brought to the operator's hands, and by the 1980s the field of inquiry was extended to the vascular tree.[38] To touch only briefly upon other applications (like looking at the inside of mummies, aircraft machinery, or listing developments in astrophotography or telecommunications) would need another book.

Another stretching of our visual perception was in microscopic dimensions. The limits of the optical microscope magnification were set, or rather stymied by the length of the wave length of visual light, although some ingenious tricks rendered improvements. One of them was the use of phase difference of lightwaves created by the difference in refractive index of the medium to be examined and the incident beam hitting it. Because of this (with certain ingenious additions) an interference would occur and, as Zernicke wrote in 1934, "transparent details of the object . . . (would) appear as differences of intensity in the image."[39] The "phase contrast microscope" was first produced commercially in the Zeiss factory, and it was widely used to observe live cells after the First World War. Another technical arrangement separated two beams of light, then recombined them to give optical interference (Smith 1947), the so-called interference microscope that further increased the acuity of observation. Additional refinements were made possible with examination in ultraviolet light.

In 1924 the Frenchman de Broglie suggested that electrons could also be regarded as waves. Busch in 1926 postulated that a "magnetic coil which focused the electron beam could be regarded as analogous to an optical lens."[40] In the early 1930s Knoll and Ruska and von Borries in Berlin constructed a microscope in which electrons instead of light rushed toward the specimen; and electromagnets instead of glass directed the electron beam. Eventually magnification up to ten thousand times was reached. What a difference: nearly three hundred years needed to perfect the optical microscope, and now in a short decade the pinnacle of previous achievements was surpassed with magnifications five to six times as high. In the 1950s results further improved. Resolution (distinction of separate structures) increased, and points to be identified came down from one hundred Angstroms to twenty-five, then five, and finally three. The highest resolution optical microscopes could muster was very little with regard to the cell cytoplasm or the nucleus, whereas the electron microscope demonstrated membrane systems, mitochondria, lysosomes, and endoplasmic reticulum—things previously unseen.

The scanning electron microscope represented further advance. When a thin layer of metal was applied to the surface of the specimen, a remarkably beautiful and realistic three-dimensional image could be obtained. Magnifications reached fifty thousand or more times the original dimensions, compared to an enlargement of a foot to double the height of the Himalaya, or one mile pulled to the length of one and a half times the circumference of the earth. The limitation of all electron-microscopes is that they have to work in a vacuum; consequently, living cells cannot be examined. Nevertheless, medicine today can see macromolecules, whereas in the seventeenth century researchers were happy to visualize red blood cells.

Using X rays to show microstructures came to mind early after X rays were discovered, and the first aim was to try to enlarge anything that researchers could lay their hands upon. In Paris, Goby in 1913 took pictures of foraminifera, a foot of a lizard with magnification up to seventeen times.[41] This soon was improved in England to forty times. The French, however, were in the forefront in this field, with Paul Lamarque and others in the mid-1930s reaching levels previously undreamed of.[42] By the 1940s microradiography was being accepted and valued in metallurgy and botanical studies, but the real breakthrough came with the "crush syndrome." Trueta and his group made a study of the unfortunate victims of the London air raids during the war, when building debris crushed the victims' limbs, compressing them with ensuing renal damage. Barklay, the radiologist of the team, made superb magnifications of tiny vessels by injecting contrast material into them; with that process he was able to show even ramifications in the glomeruli.[43] Incidentally, the first vascular magnifications with X rays were made by the Russians Grechishkin and Prives in 1935.[44] Following Barklay's example, several investigators took up the study of the finer vascular supply, and in the 1960s of all things magnified microangiography seemed best suitable to X-ray microscopy.[45]

Although X-ray microscopy was widely used on autopsy material, live objects could be enlarged only twofold. Already in 1928 Vallebona in Italy achieved direct radiographic enlargement, but it took the development of fine focus (0.3 mm) X-ray tubes to get decent pictures.[46] The Dutch Philips Company produced the first of such tubes in 1943; consequently, it was the Dutch who reaped the victory.[47] Van der Plaats was the leader in the early 1950s, but the Japanese Komiyama followed suit, and radiologists all over the world were experimenting with magnification radiography.[48] With miniaturization of the focal spot down to 0.03 mm, magnifications up to ten to twenty times were reached in the 1960s.[49] For routine work, however, twofold magnification became the standard. Bones, joints, pulmonary nodules, teeth, angiography, and calcification in the female breast (so crucial in the search for carcinoma) proved to be the most promising for direct enlargement of radiographs, strong contrast being the prerequisite.[50]

Good contrast was the determinant of producing good discrimination of tissues or organs against the background or against each other. As long as one had high atomic number elements to deal with—like Ca in bones or I or Ba as introducible material into cavities or vessels—one fared well. However, there were great difficulties in the soft tissues, which lacked high atomic number elements. A muscle was not distinguished from its neighbor, and the structures of the pelvis could not be identified unless they contained some contrast either introduced from the outside, or gas. The retroperitoneum and mediastinum were seen as conglomeration of components that could not be identified individually. And how important it would have been to locate breast tumors, which cause thirty-eight thousand deaths each year in the United States.

One first had to become acquainted with the appearance of normal conditions and then disease in the breast. In 1913 Salomon, the Berlin surgeon, dealt with operated breast specimens and correlated the X-ray images with their microscopic findings of some three thousand mastectomies.[51] His observations became the springboard for all further studies, but he still had to satisfy himself with the limitations of the "gas tubes." In 1930 Warren of Rochester, New York, published his findings in 119 cases of live mammography. His stereoscopic views claimed a 95 percent diagnostic accuracy—an enviable figure, but one that could not be duplicated by other investigators.[52] His method fell into disrepute.

Other studies introduced contrast materials to visualize the lactiferous ducts, but no processes seemed promising until Leborgne from Uruguay, in 1949, used low kilovoltage to point out calcifications in many malignant tumors, especially in intraductal carcinoma. He showed that their presence, if evaluated prudently, could be pathognomonic.[53] He also clarified certain characteristics of malignancies.

Numerous articles of Gershon-Cohen from New York called attention to the practical importance of mammography, but it was the thousand cases of Egan from Houston in 1960 that popularized mammography.[54] Egan's fine-grained industrial film was one of the secrets of his superior images. A few years later Gros in Strasbourg exchanged tungsten for molybdenum in the X-ray tube and worked with a finer focal spot than previously. These technical advances finalized the basis for the method we use today, giving finer details and showing smaller calcifications than ever before.[55] The xerography or xero-mammography of Gould for a while competed with film-screen mammography because enhancement of contours and more prominent demonstration of calcifications are appealing.[56] On the other hand, at least five times higher radiation exposure turned most radiologists to film-screen mammography, especially as the method gained much refinement. Other methods were sometimes promoted, including thermography and transillumination. Only ultrasound is regarded today as an improvement, having the advantage of not employing radiation. But ultrasound experienced full fruition only in the 1970s.

Ultrasonography started its curriculum in Pierre Curie's laboratory. With his brother Jacques, Pierre observed that an electric current appeared across crystals of quartz when they compressed them. Turning the sequence around: deformity of the crystals resulted when charged by rapidly changing electrical current. This "piezo-electric phenomenon" induced the brothers to design a refined electrometer that could measure low-intensity electric currents with great accuracy.[57] Years later, when Paul Langevin joined Pierre Curie in the Sorbonne, he was impressed with the piezo-electric phenomenon, but it took another fourteen years before he started to work in a crucial practical application: locating German submarines in the First World War. The principle Langevin worked with was simple enough: to send high-frequency sound waves beyond what could be heard by our ears (ultrasound) to the submarine target where some of them would be absorbed, some would be bounced back, and this echo could be picked up (sound navigation ranging: sonar). The closer the rebounding object, the sooner the echo would return, like the "backpacker's technique"— said Schueler, an expert in the field—checking the distance of the opposite wall of the canyon.[58] The concept was ingenious, but Langevin did not see its intended application: the war was over before his device could be used.

The first to send sound waves through the skull for diagnostic purposes was the Hungarian Benedek, around 1930. He first applied mechanical knocks on the skull, changing their frequency and intensity with an electrically operated device; then he picked up the sound on the opposite side of the skull and was able in certain instances to make the diagnosis of hydrocephalus and brain tumors. His "craniosonoscopy" method did not become internationally known. Anyway, it used low-frequency audible sound waves.[59]

The first to employ high-frequency ultrasound for medical purposes was an Austrian physician, Dussik, who tried to outline the cerebral ventricles on the premise that at the edges of the fluid-filled compartments the absorption of ultrasound would be different from that which tissues would show. Unfortunately, bones of the skull proved to be more absorbing than ventricular walls, so the idea of "hyper-phonography" of the brain fell through.[60]

Ultrasonography was not widely utilized in medicine until tracing the absorption of the waves was abandoned in favor of picking up echoes. An intern, Howry, became interested in ultrasonic visualization of tissues as early as 1947, and he wisely affiliated himself with the engineer Bliss and started experimentation with surplus Navy sonar equipment. The submarine aspect of the project was so persuasive that he immersed his subjects first in a laundry tub, then in a B-29 gun turret he called a "scanning tank"

(1952). Patients were submerged up to their necks to take readings.[61] Howry and Bliss were able to demonstrate anatomical details of the breast, as well as gallstones, and later carotid arteries, jugular veins, and abscess of the liver, among other things.[62]

In the University of Lund, Sweden, the cardiologist Edler got together with the physicist Hertz in the canteen (a frequent spawning ground of scientific thought), and they borrowed an ultrasonic instrument from the Malmö shipyard to check cardiac wall movements, valves in patients, and in some cases they used it in open-heart surgery.[63] In the United States, Satomura in 1957 introduced the Doppler effect to check cardiac wall motion. The reflected waves had higher frequency when the wall moved toward the transducer and lower frequency if the wall moved away.[64]

About the same time Leksell, a Swede, succeeded in tracing midline displacement in brain pathology, which started the method of echo-encephalography.[65] Mundt and Hughes studied the eye with ultrasound in 1956, and in 1958 Donald in Glasgow applied ultrasonics to obstetrics.[66] In a few years Donald improved his technique by moving the ultrasonic device along the skin, employing a thin oil layer between the two.[67]

By the end of the 1960s many of the body's regions were explored with ultrasound. The technology changed rapidly from investigator to investigator, as none of the employed techniques seemed satisfactory. No matter how the approach was changed with different types of water bath, or with mechanical or electronic systems coupled with photography or other recording modalities, the drawback was always that the results were shown in the "bistable mode," an image that registered all echoes above a given intensity with the same brightness, but nothing at all below a certain threshold.[68] The struggle with these problems characterized the examinations throughout the 1960s. It would have been useful to have equipment showing different grades of returning intensity of speed of echoes, but it was not available at the time.

To pursue the elusive lymphatic channels, Kinmouth from England, after numerous animal experiments and human trials, came up with a clinically useful approach in 1955: methylene blue was injected between two toes, subcutaneously rendering the nimble, fragile lymph vessels visible on the dorsum of the foot.[69]

This enabled radiologists to locate the vessels and inject contrast material into them. The slow flow of the lymph then carried the contrast material through the lymph vessels to the lymph nodes, all the way up to the pelvic and para-aortic nodes, revealing eventual pathology in them. Particularly malignant metastases could be diagnosed, and that not only assisted in determining the treatment field for radiation therapy but also showed the full extension of the spreading disease for chemotherapy evaluation. The method was used for a time in the United States but was not popular because it was so time consuming.[70] When CT scanning became available, the procedure was happily abandoned.

The possibilities of technology seemed to have been exhausted for X-ray examinations as well as for nuclear medicine and ultrasound. Then help came from an unexpected corner seemingly not closely related to imaging: mathematics.

9

A Great Leap from Tiny Chips: Computerization, 1960s and 1970s

IN 1917 the Austrian mathematician J. H. Radon published the results of his studies showing that the image of a three-dimensional object could be reconstructed from an infinite number of two-dimensional projections.[1] His work concerned astrophysics, however, not medical imaging. He could not have known that some fifty years later his calculations would lay the mathematical foundation for a great advancement in diagnostic radiology.

In the 1950s, Allan MacLeod Cormack, a Cape Town physicist, started to think about the question of how one could calculate absorption in different tissues inside the body. His project concerned the improvement of radiation therapy planning. If he knew the composition of tissues in the volume irradiated, he could calculate the absorption of the radiation dose. He worked with disks of aluminum and wood, took readings of gamma radiation data from many angles, and made his mathematical calculations. Unaware of Radon's work many years earlier, he considered this project a sideline, not serious physics—as he later recalled. In 1957, when offered an opportunity to further his studies in Boston, he ended up in the physics department of Tufts University, where he continued his earlier experiments. He embedded two aluminum objects asymmetrically into lucite to simulate tumors in the skull. His calculations and the concept of detecting tissues in the body with absorption difference from the surrounding tissues were not published in a medical journal where they could have attracted interest, but in the *Journal of Applied Physics* in 1963 and 1964. Physicists who read the report were not especially interested, and he received only two or three requests for reprints. Cormack was satisfied that he had solved the mathematical problem, but he did not carry his findings any further.[2]

Early computers in the 1940s and 1950s were mainly utilized for ballistic missile calculations by the United States Army or the space program. The brilliant mathematician who was instrumental in designing the first "modern" computers, von Neumann, emphasized in one of his articles that "technology has largely replaced geography as the main element in national power" and that "the advantage in war and international politics belongs to the nation that sets the pace in technological development."[3] With the defense-oriented programs, computers received substantial financial support and publicity.

With almost unlimited subsidies, computers became more sophisticated and efficient every passing year. For example, the IBM 1955 model could handle five thousand instructions, the 1959 model close to a million, and the 1964 operating system several million.[4] In the 1960s, miniaturized vacuum tubes were replaced by silicone transistors and magnetic tapes by discs; these innovations increased processing speed dramatically. The size of computers came down from mammoth machines requiring a space of one thousand square feet to desk-size models. Prices fell from several hundred thousand dollars to a couple of thousand dollars or less. No wonder that manufacturers, insurance companies, banks, and other commercial enterprises used them extensively for billing and payroll computations, airline reservations, meteorological calculations, and a host of administrative functions. Business and science jumped at the opportunities offered by computers. Even games started to be devised for them; the first chess program was worked out in 1952 by Turing, one of the great computer designers.

The role of the computer in human enterprise became evident;

witness to this was the letter written in 1976 by French President Giscard d'Estaing to Inspector General Simon Nora: "The applications of the computer have developed to such an extent that the economic and social organization of our society and our way of life may well be transformed as a result."[5] A similar fundamental influence upon mankind occurred in the fifteenth century with another technical innovation: the printing press. When it became available, printing companies grew like mushrooms, publishing hundreds of books yearly, changing society's thinking on everything. Repetition of the false beliefs and superstitions of the Middle Ages faded; a new era came into being. In the latter half of the twentieth century, computers made exploration of the solar system possible, gave new form to finances, and affected social development, work, education, and entertainment. How could medicine stay unaffected by this general transformation?

The medical profession also showed some interest in computers but generally regarded them as "ancillary," useful in data analysis for assessing diagnostic probabilities based upon symptoms, for retrieval of reports, and for administrative and library activities or bookkeeping.[6] There was talk of using computers to distinguish the normal from the abnormal in radiographs automatically—that was the ultimate that the medical profession was reaching for.[7] To this date, automated diagnosis on the basis of image analysis by computers has not worked out. Whereas engineering and computer science deals with well-defined, precisely reproducible factors, human anatomy is extremely variable. The author of this section was involved with advising a graduate student in computer science whose research project for a master's degree involved writing a computer program that would analyze an image of the brain to determine the presence of a subdural hematoma.[8] Although the student ultimately received his degree, the problem remained unsolved. It taught us all a lesson of how complicated such a project can be.

What else computers could possibly contribute in a branch of medicine dealing with imaging was quite uncertain until a man with imagination and competence in computer design and operation came on the scene: Godfrey Newbold Hounsfield.

Hounsfield was born in Newark, England, in 1919. Even as a

child he had his own workshop and was interested in how things worked. He received training in radio communications and served in the Royal Air Force during World War II. After the war he studied electrical and mechanical engineering. Upon graduation in 1951 he joined EMI Central Research Laboratories in London, a large electronics firm specializing in entertainment—producing phonograph records and movie films, sponsoring social clubs and dance halls, and launching the career of the Beatles. As project engineer for the first EMI Digital Equipment Corporation (DEC) solid-state computer (the first built in England), Hounsfield performed research on thin film, large-capacity memory storage and became thoroughly familiar with the intricacies of computer science.[9] Unaware of Cormack's work, he turned his attention to the problem of how an object hidden in a box could be identified by observations made from outside the box. It occurred to him in 1967 that the object could be recognized by sending a pencil-size beam of radiation through the box from multiple angles and measuring the change in the absorption of radiation caused by the hidden object. He reasoned that if such data were collected, with the help of a computer, from enough angles, the observer could determine the size and shape of the hidden object. The concept was reminiscent of conventional tomography: to see things not in the projection of the whole body, but in a narrow slice "cut" through it. The big difference was that while in conventional X-ray tomography much of the radiation exposure was wasted in areas not utilized for image production, the computerized process would characterize the target as well as the surrounding tissues. Hounsfield could declare: "I devised a system that would use 100% (of the data)."[10]

The first experiments were conducted with a very simple setup: an object was immersed in a "water box" on top of an old lathe-bed.[11] Radiation was derived initially from a gamma-ray source, and scanning lasted nine days. The data were then processed on a mainframe computer, and the calculations took two and one-half hours. The results were promising so he continued. The substitution of an X-ray tube for the gamma-ray source reduced the scanning time to minutes. The addition of an on-site minicomputer significantly shortened the time of data processing. The different absorption characteristics were represented by numerical figures, and they showed recognizably varying numbers. Eventually, he experimented with pig and cow brains as well as a human specimen obtained from a hospital museum. Hounsfield became acquainted with neuroradiologist James Ambrose and with radiologist Louis Kreel, whose interest lay in abdominal radiology. Together they started to work on patients with clinical problems.

The first patient, a woman with a suspected brain lesion, was examined in 1972.[12] By that time significant improvements of the instrument had been made. During the first experimental prototype of the scanner, an animal brain was immersed in water and rotated on the lathe in a fixed radiation beam. That method was not practical when examining live human subjects. The new design kept the patient fixed and moved the X-ray tube. Instead of immersing the patient's head in water, a tight-fitting rubber bag filled with water surrounded the head and served as the water bath. Scanning took about four minutes per slice, and the images showed a circular cyst. White matter, grey matter, and ventricles could be recognized. Hounsfield and the radiologists were jubilant.

Building on their success, they made further modifications that allowed the thousands of readings from the detectors to be fed into a dedicated minicomputer. Initially the data were presented as a printout of thousands of numbers on a sheet of paper. The numbers represented relative density to X rays of a mosaic of small volumes (pixels) of the tissue making up the slice. The initial instrument presented the data as a layout (matrix) of 80 x 80 (6,400) numbers. Although the engineers were satisfied with data printed out as numbers, physicians preferred to view them as images. Soon they converted the computed numerical data into a mosaic of grey tones, the shade of which was proportional to the absorption coefficient of the small volume of tissue represented by each pixel. The relatively large size of the pixels (1.5 mm x 1.5 mm) of the first commercially available scanner gave the appearance of a mosaic or a Mexican rug.[13] Some early models of other manufacturers even used color to represent differences in tissue density.

The beauty of the instrument was that it could detect small variations of absorption coefficients—and thus normal and pathological structures in the living body—far better than conventional X-ray equipment could. The absorption coefficient of water was arbitrarily taken as 0, that of air as -500, and of dense bone as +500 units. The scale was later changed to -1,000 to +1,000 units, subsequently named Hounsfield units.[14] Also, one could concentrate on a short segment of the scale (window), selecting the parameters that demonstrated the questionable tissue most promisingly.[15] Although the Hounsfield number of a tissue is helpful in identifying it, there is enough of an overlap among tissues to make identification on the basis of density numbers alone insufficient. Morphology, along with density, remains necessary for interpretation of an image.

The first article of Hounsfield and Ambrose about the use of computed tomography of the brain appeared in the *British Journal of Radiology* in 1973.[16] It was a sensation, and soon Hounsfield gave a talk about the scanner to invited guests from all over the world. An American engineer quite excitedly rushed to him, asking how long it would take for the Americans to start building such a machine. Hounsfield looked at his wristwatch and answered: "About 20 minutes, because it will take this time for you to rush to the phone and call up the press and the manufacturers." As a matter of fact, Hounsfield's team chose the unpretentious Atkinson Morley Hospital in Wimbledon to conduct the initial studies, bypassing the prestigious university hospitals in order to avoid interfering news media and scientific scavengers.[17]

The new instrument and its product needed a name. The early users referred to it as the EMI scanner, after its manufacturer. Soon, however, other companies started producing their own versions. The terms *computer assisted tomography* (CAT scan), *computerized axial tomography,* and *computerized axial transverse tomography* (CATT scan) became popular for a while owing to the fact that images were obtained in the transverse axial (cross-sectional) plane, even though the procedure had nothing to do with furry felines. At the First International Symposium on Computerized Axial Tomography, held at the Montreal Neurological Institute in the spring of 1974, several designations were considered. After some discussion the term *computed tomography* (CT scanning, or simply CT) was agreed upon. *Tomography* is a well-accepted term for body section imaging, and *computed* indicates that the image is generated by computer.

CT scanning not only completely revolutionized neuroradiology but had far-reaching influence upon the whole health care industry.[18] The high cost of the instrument (about a million dollars) was blamed for the escalating cost of medical care in the late 1970s and the 1980s. Sometimes it was referred to derisively as the doctors' toy. In reality it replaced many invasive and expensive diagnostic procedures. Whereas the workup of a patient suspected of having a brain lesion took as much as a week of in-hospital investigation prior to CT, a single outpatient CT scan provided as much information at less expense, thereby creating many empty hospital beds. The CT scan was a significant factor in shifting health care from the hospital to the outpatient setting.[19] Everyone interested in brain pathology jumped on the bandwagon, and radiological journals were filled with thousands and thousands of pages about important or not-so-important minutiae of the brain.

Finally, the brain was visualized. The painful, difficult, and sometimes dangerous pneumoencephalography and ventriculography, with frequently questionable results, were procedures of the past. Isotope studies had potentials, but the images lacked the resolution that CT scans could provide. Angiograms, no matter how elegant and important to show the arterial and venous systems, were frequently not specific or informative enough. They demonstrated only the "plumbing system of the house, not the building and inside proper." Previously, the possibility of distinguishing cerebral nuclei, grey and white matter, and stroke versus hemorrhage in tumor was considered unachievable.

The design of the initial EMI scanner permitted examination of the head only. It became obvious, however, that by constructing a larger instrument, the entire body could be examined. Robert Ledley, an American scientist, built the first whole-body scanner. Although he received his doctorate in dentistry, Ledley was more interested in electrical engineering and pursued further studies in that field. An innovative thinker by nature, he designed several pieces of automated equipment for laboratory use. He and his team worked on projects involving computer pattern recognition in the 1960s and 1970s. He plunged into CT scanning with great vigor and installed his prototype scanner at the Georgetown University Medical Center in February 1974. His instrument was named the automated computerized transverse axial (ACTA) scanner.[20] It incorporated several refinements compared to Hounsfield's original instrument. For example, his model did not require a water bath, and it provided an image of 160 x 160 matrix. These advances were, in turn, later incorporated into the EMI scanner. In contrast to Hounsfield, Ledley did not have the resources of a large corporation behind him. As president of the National Biomedical Research Foundation at Georgetown University, he hoped that his invention would be bought by a commercial firm so that the proceeds of the sale could finance his next project. About a year later, the Pfitzer Corporation did just that. Soon other manufacturers—American, European, and Japanese—entered the field just as Hounsfield had predicted; within a few years, EMI discontinued its manufacture of CT scanners. Ledley's prototype scanner is now at the Smithsonian Institution, underscoring its importance in the history of medical imaging.

In 1972 the prestigious MacRobert Award, often cited as the engineering equivalent of the Nobel Prize, was presented to Godfrey Hounsfield and EMI for the invention of the scanner that brought national prestige and income to the United Kingdom. In 1979 Cormack and Hounsfield shared the Nobel Prize in Medicine for their pioneering work on computed tomography. It was an honor richly deserved, for their contribution to modern medical imaging is second only to Roentgen's discovery. An interesting sidelight is that neither Cormack nor Hounsfield held a doctorate in his field.

Within a decade CT scanning became widely accepted as a diagnostic tool for a variety of disease processes. CT's greatest impact has been on neuroradiology. Such painful and occasionally hazardous invasive procedures as ventriculography and pneumoencephalography were replaced by this new noninvasive approach, which permitted visualization of the brain with far better detail. The mystique of the neuroradiologist—able to conjure an image of the brain from small collections of air on a pneumoencephalogram—diminished somewhat, as every radiologist (indeed, every physician) believed, rightly or wrongly, that he could do just as well, using the superior resolution of the CT scanner. The role of cerebral angiography also changed as it became confined largely to the investigation of vascular lesions. In the spine, CT provided superior images of the bony structures, but the visualization of the spinal cord had to await further developments. With subsequent improvement of resolution, CT became an important method in the diagnosis of herniated intervertebral disc, especially in the lumbar area, with the result that myelography had to be performed rather rarely.[21]

In the chest CT permitted improved visualization of smaller lesions, particularly those close to the chest wall, than was possible on the routine chest X ray. Lesions in the mediastinum became visible, especially if vascular structures were enhanced by intravenous contrast material. Pneumomediastinum—used in previous decades to try to outline different structures otherwise fused with each other on routine chest X rays—was made obsolete by CT, which was able to identify them separately, thereby avoiding the cumbersome injection of air or CO_2 into the mediastinum.

The deep-seated organs of the abdomen—pancreas, adrenal glands, prostate, and para-aortic lymph nodes—were seen clearly for the first time in a noninvasive way. Disease processes in these areas hitherto often required exploratory surgery.

In the musculoskeletal system, the depiction of soft-tissue structures was a novelty, whereas most of the time bone lesions were only adequately seen on conventional films, by now neglected by the CT enthusiasts quite frequently. Seeing the extent of soft-tissue invasion of a bone tumor, or vice versa, was made possible. In the case of spinal injury the visualization of the full extent of bony injury and intrusion of fragments into the spinal canal resulted in better care for those patients.

Virtually all specialties of medicine benefitted from improved visual perception of normal and abnormal tissues and organs by the CT scanner. In 1985 a fractured tooth was successfully shown on a CT scan that otherwise could not have been perceived, thus extending its benefits to dentistry.[22]

It was soon realized that the intravenous injection or oral ingestion of contrast materials prior to scanning, as in other radiological procedures, would further aid in the evaluation of the images. Contrast materials contain iodine, making vascular or other structures identifiable in the scan. "Contrast enhancement" is widely used in CT scanning in our day.

In the late 1970s, researchers at the Mayo Clinic built a super CT scanner employing twenty-eight X-ray tubes for rapid imaging of the whole body. The super scanner was capable of acquiring data for 240 contiguous slices in as little as ten milliseconds. Although the monstrous instrument, named Dynamic Spacial Reconstructor (DSR), was functional, it was expensive and cumbersome and no other such machine was built.

The basic design of the CT scanner changed very little into the 1980s, although there were many improvements in image quality. From the relatively crude 80 x 80 matrix of the first commercial EMI scanner, to the 512 x 512 matrix of the instruments of the late 1980s, it was as if someone had turned on a bright light in a previously dimly lit room. Scanning time was shortened to a matter of seconds and, for one model, to even less than a second. Normal and abnormal organs and tissues were presented in exquisite detail, enabling the well-trained specialist to make the diagnosis faster, more accurately, and with more confidence than ever before. Computed tomography and other new imaging modalities largely replaced exploratory surgery. This, in turn, resulted in shortened hospital stays or no hospitalization at all. Nothing, however—not even the most sophisticated computers—has replaced the well-trained experienced human being who interprets the images produced by the scanner.

The 1970s brought about other developments in medical terminology, largely made possible by rapid developments in computer technology. Ultrasonography was one of the major beneficiaries. Until the 1970s, imaging with sound waves above the range perceived by the human ear (ultrasound) struggled with a technique known as the "bistable mode," which was able to depict areas from which a signal was either received or not received at all, nothing in between regardless of the frequency or penetration power of the beam of sound. Compound scanning—directing the transducer from different angles—did eliminate some of the drawbacks of single scanning, but the inability to distinguish between different tissues while showing echoes from all of them limited the usefulness of ultrasound. Then in 1972 came an idea from the Australian Kossoff, who found that photographic film would show shades of grey depending upon the strength of the reverberated beam.[23]

The human eye can distinguish without difficulty ten or twelve shades of grey. Registering twelve grades of difference according to the characteristics of the echo helped the ultrasound machine distinguish the subtle variations of reverberated echoes of various tissues, and even between normal and abnormal states of organs. The favorites to depict were those reminiscent of the origins of ultrasonics: the submarines, something solid floating in water. What could be closer to this physical arrangement than a fetus floating in amniotic fluid, or gallstones in bile, or cardiac valves and wall movements, or the lens of the eye, or a foreign body in the vitreous? With grey scale, scanning the placenta could be well-demonstrated with even a hint as to its maturity. And if liquids next to solids were easy to observe, cysts became cherished targets. All those possibilities were shown by Kossoff and his associates (Garrett, Carpenter, and others). Cysts in the thyroid, breast, and kidneys could be identified without the intervention of needle puncture.[24] Consequently, the decade saw increasing use of ultrasound scanning. In the early 1980s improved electronics and transducers allowed visualization of the area examined not on photographic film or on the oscillograph but right then and there—in real time on a video screen. Examination took less time; moreover, vessels could be followed easily, respiration did not interfere, and less skill was required of the examiner than in the older B-scan variety.

As electronics and retrieval of data were computerized, a great debate started to surface in ultrasound technology: Should the data be handled with analogue or digital equipment? Within a short time the digital camp reaped victory. It would be interesting to quote those who first started real time and the proponents of digitization. No single person can be pinpointed any longer, however. The more complicated the technology becomes, the more experts are needed, especially in the clinical setting. Physicists, electrical engineers, chemists, surgeons, radiologists, and groups compete with each other in multiple corners of the world—not to speak of rival manufacturing companies. Scientific articles nowadays have five or six authors, frequently ten or more, sometimes as many as twenty. Increasingly, results are not reached by individuals but tend to be institutional or global achievements of a specific era or area.

Ultrasound is also capable of depicting movement based on the Doppler principle, which was utilized in imaging cardiac wall motion by the Japanese Satomura in 1955.[25] In those days neither grey scale nor real time ultrasound were available, and the uncertainties with continuous wave instrumentation and artifacts prevented the method from becoming popular.[26] Then came the innovation that sent bursts of ultrasound at regular intervals through tissues, eliminating some of the problems. This was only possible when the so-called duplex scanners became available in the late 1970s. They combined pulsed echoes with real time systems and were able to show flow characteristics in vessels as well as tissues and plaques in arteries, making the approach practical and attractive.[27]

Icing on the cake was the introduction of color by the Japanese in the early 1980s.[28] Color gained popular acclaim in cardiac diagnostics as well as evaluation of the peripheral circulation.[29] The vivid, eye-catching color made diagnosticians, who were accustomed to dull shades of grey, spellbound.

Another victory for computers was yet another type of examination. Certain radioactive isotopes decay by emitting a positron. After traveling a very short distance, this positively charged particle collides with a negatively charged electron. The resulting reaction ("annihilation reaction") results in two high-energy photons traveling in exactly the opposite direction. The products of the annihilation reaction can be detected and quantitated with great accuracy using paired detectors opposite each other on either side of the object being scanned. Although such scanners were in use in the 1960s, their usefulness was greatly facilitated by the addition of a computer to analyze the data as is done in computed tomography. The computerized instrument, which resembles a CT scanner, is named a positron emission tomography, or PET scanner.[30]

Whereas the CT scanner uses an external X-ray beam generated by an X-ray tube, the PET scanner utilizes radiation emitted by the positron-emitting isotope administered internally to the patient. It so happens that the radioactive isotopes of carbon (C-11), nitrogen (N-13), oxygen (O-15), and fluorine (F-18) are all positron emitters. Carbon, nitrogen, and oxygen are components of most metabolically active compounds in the body and are thus ideal agents to study physiological processes in vivo. Fluorine can be tagged to other elements to study their metabolic pathways. As a group, positron-emitting isotopes have one thing in common: They have very short half lives, measured in minutes. While the short half life results in low radiation exposure to the patient, it makes these substances expensive and difficult to work with. They must be produced in a cyclotron in close proximity to the PET scanner. Recent advances of miniaturization in cyclotron design made it possible to manufacture small units for the specific purpose of producing radiopharmaceuticals for the PET scanner.

Impressive studies have been conducted on the functioning human brain with the use of PET. For example, the PET scan could detect increased metabolic activity of the occipital cortex, the area of the brain related to vision, on patients who were given oxygen-15 labeled glucose and told to concentrate on looking at a picture. Such metabolic activity cannot only be seen but quantitated with great accuracy. For the first time, localized metabolic aberrations have been detected in specific areas of the brain, raising hope that PET will lead to improved understanding of some mental illnesses. Monte Buchsbaum of the University of California at Irvine found diminished glucose metabolism in the frontal lobes of schizophrenics. In 1985, a man stood before a court, accused of having killed four members of his family. Although he had been previously diagnosed a schizophrenic, under California law the defense found insanity difficult to prove. Buchsbaum's testimony regarding the findings on PET scan of reduced frontal lobe activity was accepted by the court as objective evidence of mental illness, the first time that such evidence was admitted.[31] Similarly, patients suffering from Alzheimer's disease showed abnormal metabolic activity throughout the brain. PET scanning promises to be useful in the evaluation of efficacy of treatment of disorders of the brain and in the evaluation of the viability of the heart muscle of patients with coronary insufficiency. It was found that the PET scan is a far better predictor of patient response to revascularization procedures than other available techniques. Finally, PET scanning is able to show effectiveness of chemotherapy of certain tumors by analyzing their metabolic activity. Thus, the treatment protocol may be adjusted for maximum benefit.

Single-photon emission computed tomography (SPECT) scanning also uses subatomic particles to form images. It is a refinement of radionuclide imaging using the Anger camera. Employing techniques similar to those utilized in CT scanning, SPECT scanning produces images of slices of the body, albeit with much less spacial resolution than CT. The commonly used radionuclide is Iofetamine HC1 tagged with [123]I. It is lipophilic (fat soluble) and is thus able to enter the brain through an intact blood-brain barrier. It is able to delineate viable nervous tissue and is especially helpful in the examination of patients after stroke.[32] SPECT scanning is likewise used to detect viable cardiac muscle after myocardial infarction; thus, it aids in the determination of the prognosis and in selection of patients for cardiac surgery.[33]

In terms of producing a tomographic representation of the distribution of radionuclide, SPECT and PET scanning are similar. The use of oxygen, nitrogen, and carbon isotopes in PET scanning make that procedure far more useful in metabolic research, however.

In addition to new imaging techniques, computerization has been applied to conventional X-ray images. The images are vastly improved and can be further enhanced by digital techniques, while at the same time patient exposure to ionizing radiation is reduced. For example, the radiologist viewing a single digital chest X-ray film can vary the technique of the image on the computer screen to show lung, mediastinum, or bone to better advantage without subjecting the patient to additional radiation exposure, as would be required when using conventional techniques.[34]

Computerization has been applied to angiography with spectacular results. Just prior to World War II, Ziedses des Plantes, the Dutch neuroradiologist, invented subtraction radiography.[35] Although fine detail was easier to see with his photographic technique, the procedure was laborious and time-consuming until assisted by computerization. The procedure that became known as Digital Subtraction Angiography (or DSA) was successfully accomplished at the University of Wisconsin in 1976.[36] With a computer program, the first image is reversed on the video display screen, and the subsequent images are presented as already subtracted as they are obtained. The result is vastly clearer images, obtained in a much shorter time with smaller amounts of contrast material injected. DSA is a safer procedure and in many instances can be performed on an outpatient basis. It is another example of technical innovation allowing the physician to *see* better.

With the advent of new imaging techniques and vastly improved image quality, the radiologist became an important member of the medical team. No longer was the radiologist only a consultant, but he or she became increasingly involved with direct patient care, establishing the field that became known as interventional radiology.[37] Using intravascular catheters under direct fluoroscopic control, radiologists could not only open narrowed or even occluded blood vessels but could close off such unwanted vascular structures as aneurysms, vascular fistulas, and malformations. Radiologists have learned to use catheters for removal of stones from the urinary and biliary tracts and for draining abscesses percutaneously, obviating the need for surgery.

As a result, another new term has entered medical terminology: turf battle. As radiologists with their newly expanded visual capabilities broadened also the scope of their involvement in patient care, it was often at the expense of other medical and surgical specialties. Radiology as a specialty shed its image as a group of physicians working in dimly lit backrooms of hospitals without any patient contact and became the most sought-after specialty among young physicians. Indeed in the 1970s, 1980s, and 1990s a higher percentage of medical students than ever before planned to enter radiology training. All because we can now see better with the help of computerized equipment.

So much became visualized in a short time that it seemed as though the potential of computers had exhausted medical technology. But science as well as art thrives on a basic ingredient: surprise.

10

Further Advances with Computers, 1980s and 1990s

COMPUTED TOMOGRAPHY had such an impact on medical imaging in the 1970s that it seemed nothing as spectacular could be produced again in the near future. Then an unexpected development surfaced in the very years when CT scanning dominated diagnostics. It came from a quite different angle: not ionizing radiation, as X rays or gamma rays, but magnetic forces.

In the 1920s, when Planck's quantum theory and Bohr's model of the atom were the talk of the day, one of the latter's assistants, the Austrian Wolfgang Pauli, realized that the axis of the orbital motion of electrons in the atom could be influenced by an externally applied magnetic field.[1] Somewhat later Isidor Rabi of the United States observed that the nucleus of the atom, which is a miniature magnet, spins also and the spin may be influenced by a strong magnetic field.[2]

Another fifteen years passed before Edward M. Purcell of Harvard University and the Swiss-born Felix Bloch, conducting his experiments at Stanford University, made important but independent discoveries in that field. Unaware of each other's efforts, in the 1940s they began measuring the nuclear magnetic moment using the same approach. Under normal circumstances the rotational axes of atomic nuclei are aligned in a random fashion.

Purcell and Bloch found that when they placed an element into a strong magnetic field, its group of nuclei began to precess (wobble) and align in a certain direction relative to the magnetic field.[3]

When a radio frequency was also applied, the axis of rotation of the atomic nuclei atoms changed. As soon as the radio frequency wave was turned off, the atomic nuclei resumed their previous orientation.[4] The time required to return to the original orientation is called "relaxation time," an important characteristic of the interaction.[5] At the resonant frequency, nuclei in lower states absorb radio-frequency energy and remit it as they "relax" to the ground state. The emitted radio-frequency energy is measurable. Nuclear magnetic resonance (NMR)—reversal of the energy—is a characteristic of a particular nucleus in a particular magnetic and chemical environment. Because NMR can be determined with great precision, the procedure is effective for chemical analysis in liquids as well as solids.[6] Although Purcell and Bloch worked independently and at opposite coasts of the United States, they published their results in the same year of 1946 in successive issues of the journal *Science*. In 1952 they shared the Nobel Prize for Physics.

In the 1950s and 1960s, NMR gained wide acceptance as a nondestructive analytical method in chemistry and biochemistry when measurements of relaxation times were made on chemical samples (NMR spectroscopy). NMR involved no imaging. The instruments employed small chambers, centimeters or even millimeters in diameter, into which samples were inserted. Toward the end of the 1960s, work began to apply NMR to the examination of live animal organisms, but it took years of diligent effort to reach higher levels of accomplishment.

Several biological NMR experiments examined the proton of the hydrogen atom in water; a few included sodium and phosphorus. By the late 1960s, not only liquids were tested with NMR spectroscopy signals but also muscles, a human arm, and even a live mouse.[7] These were more or less scientific curiosities until Raymond Damadian in 1971 showed that samples of malignant tumors resected from mice signaled much higher values than did normal tissues.[8] On the basis of his findings, Damadian became convinced that NMR would eventually be an important tool for diagnosing cancer. A physician on the faculty of the State University of New York Downstate Medical Center, Damadian envisioned building a magnet with a large enough bore to hold a human being.[9] The reading obtained on the machine would tell whether the patient had cancer. Damadian spent a great deal of time seeking funding for the project. Initially, he conducted his experiments on an instrument of a company manufacturing small NMR equipment. But soon he realized that the best way to achieve his objective was to build his own large-bore magnet and design it in such a way that it could produce an image of the body and localize the abnormal areas. By 1976 he called his technique for localizing the signals from the body "field-focused nuclear magnetic resonance"—or FONAR.

At about the same time, the "encoding of special coordinates by known magnetic field shapes" to map out NMR relaxation times as images occurred to Paul Lauterbur, a chemist.[10] He decided to work out the mathematical calculations to do it. He first encountered NMR when he was drafted into the United States Army during the Korean War and was assigned to the Army Chemical Center in Englewood, Maryland, where he worked with such an instrument. When he returned to civilian life, he obtained a Ph.D. from the University of Pittsburgh and joined the faculty of the State University of New York at Stony Brook. His main professional interest continued to be NMR. His approach for converting the NMR signals into images was similar to techniques for the reconstruction of CT images of objects from different projections, reminiscent of the approaches of Cormack and Hounsfield. Lauterbur applied the term *zeugmatography* to the process. The word is derived from the Greek *zeugma,* meaning "that which joins together."[11]

In the early 1970s Damadian and Lauterbur became involved in a fierce and often bitter competition to be the first to achieve NMR imaging. Lauterbur is generally credited with producing the first computerized image of two tiny water-filled tubes in a 5 mm tube in 1973.[12] Within a few years, however, several groups in the United States, England, Scotland, Switzerland, Japan, and elsewhere tackled the problem of obtaining images from hydrogen proton (water) NMR studies using different approaches.[13] The first successful image of a live animal (mouse) was obtained in Aberdeen,

Scotland, in 1974.[14] Encouraged by its success in the field of computed tomography, the EMI Corporation entered the competition to produce a clinical instrument. Research was carried out at Nottingham University and at Hammersmith Hospital in London.

By the early 1980s the first crude total human body NMR images were shown. In no time physicists and engineers of the major equipment manufacturers in the United States, Japan, and Europe, using substantially improved technology, produced the superb images we are accustomed to seeing nowadays. (EMI relinquished its role, selling its facilities to other manufacturers.) The only disadvantage of NMR is that it cannot be used on patients who have been implanted with magnetically sensitive foreign bodies containing iron (including nails, screws, surgical clips, or pacemakers) for fear of moving or desensitizing such elements.

From the beginning, one of the most attractive features of the new imaging technique was the absence of X ray or gamma radiation, eliminating an ever-present hazard of most of the previous imaging modalities. The new technique was safe in the examination of children and even pregnant women. Also, as bone contains little water, it did not interfere with visualization of soft tissues, as is the case with X rays, including CT scans. Stiff competition developed between the well-established CT and the newcomer, NMR imaging, especially in regards to the examination of the central nervous system.

The name of the new procedure was soon changed. The term *nuclear* carried the connotation of nuclear radiation and even the nuclear bomb. It also caused some confusion as to whether it was a nuclear medicine scan. So "nuclear" was dropped, and the new imaging technique became known as magnetic resonance imaging, or simply MRI.

In its early years of development as a clinical diagnostic instrument, MRI was hampered by efforts of governmental agencies and insurance companies to hold down the ever-increasing cost of medicine. MRI was seen as another expensive technology that threatened to bankrupt the medical care system, as CT was accused of doing a decade earlier. The fact that CT, and now MRI, greatly increased diagnostic accuracy and often obviated the need for other expensive procedures and hospital stays was not sufficiently appreciated. But doctors and patients demanded the new imaging technique, and slowly MRI took hold.

Although CT and MRI have many similarities, there are significant differences between them, and for the foreseeable future each appears to occupy its own niche in the diagnostic armamentarium.

To be sure, MRI is heavily based on superb depiction of anatomy. But for the first time, focal changes in biochemistry were also visually depicted. Alas, expectation of a machine that would simply and reliably determine if the patient had cancer did not materialize, although MRI certainly contributed significantly to medical diagnosis. At the present time MRI is based on imaging the proton (hydrogen nucleus) and its chemistry. Since hydrogen in the form of water is present throughout the body in various concentrations (the human body is 80 percent water), this allows visualization of many organs and tissues. Some success has been achieved in the imaging of the sodium atom, and there are efforts to image phosphorus and potassium, but their MR signal is many times weaker than that of hydrogen. Other atoms are not yet possible to image because of their even weaker magnetic resonance signal.

Magnetic resonance imaging techniques employ many different modes, including setting or changing the machinery in various ways (T1, T2, spin echo, flip angle three-dimensional time of flight MR, or pase contrast ciné MR, for example) to give pulse sequences singly or in combination.[15] The particular setting of the equipment determines how a lesion will appear on the resulting image. Selection of the proper factors is crucial because, while a lesion may be demonstrated in exquisite detail with one set of pulse sequences, it may be missed altogether with another. Thus, MRI is much more dependent on the skill and experience of the supervising radiologist than are other imaging procedures.

Technical advances present themselves in other areas too: helical CT and CT angiographic improvements, for example, and rotating digital subtraction angiography, which allows three-dimensional viewing of arteries. Three-dimensional viewing expands to ultrasonography; and color is widely employed with Doppler ultrasound, SPECT, and PET. But it will take years to determine which technology is best suited for each disease. The overwhelming variety of competing technologies induced the surveyors of the 1993 meeting of the Roentgen Society of North America to declare: "The sheer number and variety of sessions and presentations was bewildering and to some extent numbing."[16]

In contrast to CT, where the basic components of the scanner do not vary much from one model to another, the design of MRI scanners is subject to considerable variation. One is the strength of the magnetic field. As yet there is a great deal of difference of opinion among experts as to the ideal field strength. Expressed in Tesla (1 T = 10,000 Gauss), the unit of magnetic field strength, it ranges from 0.04 Tesla for ultra-low-field scanners to 1.5 Tesla for high-field instruments. By way of comparison, the strength of the magnetic field of a 1.5 Tesla scanner is 32,000 times that of the Earth. Many are in the mid-field range of 0.3 to 0.5 T. Most mid- and high-field units employ superconductive magnets requiring cooling by liquid helium and liquid nitrogen to achieve optimum operating temperatures. Others are resistive units, with a large electrical current to generate the necessary magnetic field. There are also permanent magnet units requiring neither supercooling nor large electric current. These, however, are in the ultra-low- to low-field range in strength. Generally, the higher the field strength, the higher the purchase and operating cost. In many applications, however, higher-field strength yields better image quality.

There is no question that MRI allows us to look into the living body to a greater extent than ever before. MRI images of the head provide exquisite detail of the anatomy of the brain as well as of other structures surrounding it. Images may be obtained in the axial, coronal, sagittal, and oblique planes, all with the patient lying in the supine position—a great advantage over CT, which can take slices only in the axial plane. Degradation of image quality due to the proximity of bone, a bane of CT images, is no problem for MRI because bones carry much less water (consequently hydrogen) than present-day machinery is aiming for. This results in preference for MRI in the diagnosis of disorders at the base of the skull as well as in the region of the face. Pituitary tumors, for example, are presented with a clarity never previously possible. Excellent depiction of focal areas of demyelination promise to further our understanding of multiple sclerosis and the dementias. With its superb depiction of the spinal cord and other contents of the spinal canal, MRI has replaced myelography in many instances and is likely to replace it entirely. Although the role of MRI in imaging of the chest and abdomen is less certain, the use of cardiac gating (limitation of image acquisition to certain segments of the cardiac cycle) eliminates motion artifacts and allows the imaging of heart chambers with enough precision and clarity that MRI might perhaps also replace angiography in the future. Computer programs now permit the viewing of the images in the "ciné" mode, simulating activity of the living, moving organ. That option is very helpful in looking at the heart and joints in motion. Other computer programs utilize the MRI data to render three-dimensional images, a spectacular achievement that is especially helpful to surgeons because it allows them to view and visually manipulate body parts from all angles preoperatively.

During MRI production the necessary radio waves are applied in brief spurts (pulses), and the resulting changes in the alignment of the hydrogen atoms are observed between such pulses. In the case of flowing blood, the volume of blood receiving the radio wave is often no longer in the volume of tissue imaged by the time the scanner is ready to observe the resulting changes. Thus, rapidly flowing blood produces no signal, or a void. Conversely, stagnant blood or blood contained in an occluded vessel does produce a signal. An appropriate computer program can thus offer quantitative as well as qualitative evaluation of blood flow. Further manipulation of the data results in an MRI angiogram, an image in which the blood vessels are seen as on a conventional radiographic angiogram, except no contrast material must be injected! Radiographic angiography with a needle or catheter inserted into the artery may become a thing of the past.

The noninvasive technique of MRI also offers great promise to the internal structures of joints, especially the knee. The menisci and cruciate and collateral ligaments are depicted with as much clarity as in textbooks of anatomy. Arthrography is being replaced by MRI in many institutions.

As revealing as the MRI images are, they can be further improved upon by contrast enhancement, as is the case with CT.[17] In this instance, however, the agent is not iodinated, but a paramagnetic substance, an element that has magnetic properties. Although many other substances have been investigated, gadolinium in the form of gadolinium DTPA is today the only widely used paramagnetic contrast agent. It causes a brighter signal in vascular structures and enters an abnormal area of the brain through a disturbed blood-brain barrier, causing a brighter signal in the abnormal tissue. It is used particularly in the evaluation of certain tumors, notably meningioma and acoustic neuroma.

As we approach the twenty-first century, MRI is still in its formative stage. New applications are reported daily, and its final role among medical imaging techniques has yet to be defined. Some predict that MRI will replace all or most X-ray-based imaging modalities. A very promising development in the use of magnetic resonance in medicine is the combination of magnetic resonance spectroscopy (MRS) with spectroscopic imaging.[18] In such a procedure, MRI will be used to localize the abnormal area, while spectroscopy will analyze the nature of the pathology in an entirely noninvasive way.

Computerization has impregnated all modalities of medical imaging, and it is unlikely that image retrieval will be unaffected. Images produced by different kinds of procedures must be preserved and stored for future use. "Hard copy" imaging uses films, and film utilizes silver containing chemicals. By the 1970s there were dire predictions that the silver supply of the world would soon be exhausted by the demands of medical imaging. And, in fact, in the mid-1970s silver prices did skyrocket but then settled back to more tolerable levels. But the message was clear: alternate means of image storage must be found.

In the 1980s another acronym appeared in the language of radiology: PACS, which stands for *picture archiving and communications system*. Computer technology permitted the digitization and storage on magnetic tape or discs, and more recently on optical discs, of the images produced in imaging departments, ultimately creating a filmless X-ray department. In such a department, elimination of film developing and handling will lessen the time spent on each examination, thereby reducing patient waiting. A side benefit of such an arrangement will be that a well-equipped physician will be able to call up a video screen not only with the radiologist's report but also with the complete X rays, nuclear scans, CT scans, MRI, and ultrasound images. At this time, such technology is prohibitively expensive. Small-scale systems are operational, however, proving that it is technically feasible. It will be well into the next century before all images will be stored digitally and be available at a moment's notice at the push of a button. The insatiable demand of physicians to *see* will force these potentials to a practical reality in the future.

Epilogue

HAVING REVIEWED THE PHASES of how we accumulated knowledge by seeing, we realize that the speed of advance has increased geometrically. We also realize that we depend more and more on data and images obtained by machinery. Almost every month some original invention stretches our knowledge; engineers and physicists experiment with ideas that broaden the possibilities of presently available equipment or lead to the creation of new equipment.

We are in the midst if a great leap. Science does not grow in a continuum but—as quanta of energy—jumps in packages. Our latest leap is achieved by computer technology. In the past we also have experienced breakthroughs. The development of the microscope, for example, shook up concepts of diseases and therapy. Roentgen's discovery almost overnight provided the first look into the living body. And both of those technical improvements had periods of slowdown, even retreat. Although most likely we will experience reduction of speed and progress, we still live through stunning advancements in machinery and procedures.

Think of miniaturization of fiber optics, which enables us to perform angioscopy with a bundle of fibers only 3.3 mm in diameter, or of fast-scan methods in MR studies, or the combination of techniques like coupling laser technology with other imaging modalities.[1] Science has just scratched the surface of the potential of positron emission tomography (PET). Here is a technique that displays the chemical binding of oxygen and glucose, the basic energy-producing chemical reaction of the brain. Have we reached the limits? Or will we continue?

If we try to make a reasonable forecast, we must realize that progress derives from many factors, but one thing is sure: both technical innovations and theoretical schemes come from individuals or groups of persons whose minds spin around the same theme. To figure out probabilities of tomorrow, we should examine the mental setup of investigators who developed new things and specify circumstances under which they were able to achieve those ends. How else can we even guess our future chances of progress? Many times extrapolation based on contemporary developments have proven to be fallacious.

In the introduction to his planned scientific treatise, Leonardo da Vinci wrote that he felt like someone who had arrived late at the village fair: all important items had been selected out; he would have to satisfy himself with leftovers.[2] He wrote that five hundred year ago! More recently young Einstein, after having written a congratulatory note to Roentgen for his discovery, remarked that it did not seem that the new rays could help "our insight into the fundamental properties of matter," a statement disproved by X-ray spectroscopy.[3] Predictions seem to give less credit to future progress than it deserves.

Should we then believe TV announcements or newspaper articles painting colorful pictures about solving the "cancer problem" with some yet-unheard-of laboratory procedure or equipment? Can we try to figure out what we can expect from further development in technology? And is technology the only solution? We cannot disregard the Nobelist Chain's (of penicillin fame) warning: "Let us not fall victim to the naive illusion that problems like cancer, mental illness, degeneration in old age . . . can be solved by bulldozer organizational methods such as were in the Manhattan [atomic bomb] project. . . . We had geniuses whose basic discoveries made its development possible—the Curies, the Rutherfords, Einsteins, Niels Bohrs and many others. In the biological field . . . these geniuses have not yet appeared, we are still waiting for them."[4]

The definition of genius is difficult, and its early recognition impossible. We are unable to investigate the genetic factors that would give the "hardware" of intelligence and personality, depending on the brain and the endocrine system.[5] The "software" of the system can be tracked down, however. We have seen that outside influences have paramount bearing upon the personalities of scientists. There is no question that education, information from other corners, and response by peers have formative power upon a person's mental development. Equally important are the economic, political, and academic systems in which the person lives. Briefly, the environment makes or breaks the talent, the chief generator of progress. The advancement of science—or lack of it—changes places in the course of history, depending on two basic factors, mental influences and money. In the third century B.C., Alexandria was the leader; in the fifteenth and sixteenth century, the Florentine and Venetian Republic; in the seventeenth and eighteenth century, England and France; in the nineteenth, Germany closed in. At the present, there is no single national leader, but the United States, Canada, Western Europe, and Japan are in the forefront.

As for the future? Russia has made advances in space technology, and scientists from China and India (working in United States labs) are claiming Nobel Prizes in physics and mathematics, showing that the brain power is there but opportunity is lacking. Watching Japan, one wonders whether Matsushita's dream could become true, that Japan will be the leader of the world in the twenty-first century. That well-known industrialist founded a school to train the best of his nation for the next century. The curriculum promotes foreign languages, including six-month studies in foreign countries.[6] But how far can technology carry our sciences, and how much have we gained up to now by seeing?

Interchange with other cultures can make us proud; at the same time we should also be humbled in our indoctrinated prejudices by acknowledging the achievements of other cultures and eras. We have seen that surroundings have a formidable power to lift or crush great scientific talent.

We are now in the fortunate position of visualizing much that we did not even hope to see in the past. Diagnostics in most instances are coming out of the shady premises of "circumstantial evidence" into the wonderland of direct evidence. We have a realistic hope that with more factual knowledge less will be left to guesswork. As we look at the rapid accumulation of exact information, we cannot escape the prediction that we will know more about our body and mind in the coming decades of the computer age, based on help from technology. As we witness this stupendous growth of medical sciences, we can claim that we are able to pinpoint the nature and origins of many of the ailments that bother us, with the help of our fantastically advanced equipment. But we have to stop for a moment.

At the end of the last century machinery was present in every physics laboratory to produce X rays, and as a matter of fact, several of the most outstanding physicists (Crookes, Lenard, Goodspeed) actually did produce them but did not realize it; only Roentgen recognized that something new had been found. All others had it at their fingertips but did not realize it. When Szentgyorgyi (of Vitamin C and actomyosin fame) had a pleasant frugal dinner of fresh fruit and raw vegetables, he wondered why the surface of the apple or the potato became dark, whereas green paprika retained its color. He reasoned that there had to be a strong reducing agent in the paprika to prevent some compounds from oxidation. At the time he was experimenting with hexuronic acid, a reducing compound, and concluded that that probably was what was present. He obtained enough material for chemical analysis—and hexuronic acid was in effect identified and proved to be vitamin C and, as such, renamed ascorbic acid.

At another time and place, Forbath, a leading pediatrician of Canada was shown emaciated Indian children in Mother Teresa's sanctuary. There, the poor little bodies were lying with hollow cheeks, limp feet, and limp arms. The doctor pointed to one of them, saying, "This child has meningitis." Mother Teresa asked why he thought that it was not a case of malnutrition, as were the others. "Because his extremities are spastic, not relaxed as the others," replied the doctor, and lumbar puncture proved he was right. All this without machinery.

A shocking realization about machinery hit us recently: computers are not as foolproof as they are professed to be. In NATO's military installations, one out of ten software fragments was found to contain errors.[7] In the medical electronic industry, twice as much computer-controlled equipment had to be recalled in 1984 than in any previous year. Our wonderful pushbutton machines apparently have to be watched with acute alertness, and everything must be observed with cool eyes, not giving credit to authority even if it be a machine.

Naturally we do need equipment, but we can do a lot on our own. We have a visual aid, sensitive to millimicrons of electromagnetic waves and differences in wavelengths that are recorded as color. We call it the eye. We have a highly efficient apparatus, taking sound waves and specifying them by frequency and penetration, called the ear. We also have a computer with more than 10 billion chips called neurons and each one of them with additional hundreds of connections, with their digital as well as analogue potential—the brain.[8] Of course we need machinery. But our personal contribution is indispensable.

We must not fall into the trap of mindlessly embracing fads. We must evaluate newer versus older technological approaches, weighing real advantage in diagnostics against cost effectiveness. Up-to-date techniques of the present might become outdated tomorrow. The traditionally important factors in caring for patients are not yet manageable by computer: understanding their habitats, their pains, their fears, their hopes, their expectations, and their full personalities. Ultimately, medical progress and the alleviation of human suffering will depend on technology as well as our human input.

Notes

Index

Notes

1. Early Beliefs about the Human Body, 4000–300 B.C.

1. N. Eldredge and I. Tattersall, *The Myths of Human Evolution* (New York: Columbia University Press, 1981), p. 151.

2. H. E. Sigerist, *Primitive and Archaic Medicine* (New York: Oxford University Press, 1955); J. A. Wilson, "Medicine in Ancient Egypt," *Bulletin of the History of Medicine* 36 (1962): 114–23; G. Majno, *The Healing Hand: Man and Wound in the Ancient World* (Cambridge, Mass.: Harvard University Press, 1975).

3. A. Castiglioni, *A History of Medicine,* trans. E. B. Krumbhaar (New York: Alfred A. Knopf, 1958), p. 57; W. Durant, *Our Oriental Heritage,* vol. 1 of *Story of Civilization* (New York: Simon and Schuster, 1963), p. 182.

4. Castiglioni, *History of Medicine,* p. 50.

5. J. H. Breasted, "The Edwin Smith Surgical Papyrus," *Bulletin of Social Medical History* 3 (1923): 58–78.

6. H. Von Staden, *Herophilus: The Art of Medicine in Early Alexandria* (New York: Cambridge University Press, 1989).

7. F. H. Garrison, *An Introduction to the History of Medicine* (Philadelphia: W. B. Saunders, 1961), p. 62; J. A. Garraty and P. Gay, *The Columbia History of the World* (New York: Harper and Row, 1984), p. 66.

8. Castiglioni, *History of Medicine,* p. 40; A. L. Oppenheim, "Man and Nature in Mesopotamian Civilization," *Dictionary of Scientific Biography* (New York: Charles Scribner and Sons, 1981), 14:645.

9. J. Preuss, *Biblisch-Talmudische Medizin* (Berlin: Karger, 1923).

10. Garrison, *History of Medicine,* p. 67.

11. F. Rosner, *Medicine in the Bible and the Talmud* (New York: Yeshiva University Press, 1977), p. 7.

12. C. Singer and E. A. Underwood, *A Short History of Medicine* (New York: Oxford University Press, 1962).

13. Castiglioni, *History of Medicine,* p. 89.

14. A. F. R. Hoernle, *Studies in the Medicine of Ancient India,* as cited in Castiglioni, *History of Medicine,* p. 95.

15. F. Capra, *The Tao of Physics* (New York: Bantam Books, 1977), p. 102.

16. Castiglioni, *History of Medicine,* p. 103.

17. W. R. Morse, *Chinese Medicine* (New York: P. B. Hoeber, 1934).

18. W. Durant, *The Life of Greece,* vol. 2 of *Story of Civilization* (New York: Simon and Schuster, 1963), p. 128.

19. G. B. Kerfeld, "Democritus," *Dictionary of Scientific Biography,* 4:30–35.

20. Von Staden, *Herophilus,* p. 141.

21. R. Joly, "Hippocrates," *Dictionary of Scientific Biography,* 6:418–33.

22. M. Neuburger, *History of Medicine,* trans. E. Playfair (London: Oxford University Press, 1925).

23. A. Krug, *Hippokrates in Heilkunst und Heilkult: Medizin in der Antike* (Munich: Beck, 1984).

24. H. Grensemann, "Die Hippokratische Schrift ueber die Heilige Krankheit," *Ars Medica* 2 (1968): 1.

25. Xenophon, *Memorabilia,* as cited in Durant, *Life of Greece,* p. 372.

26. Ibid., p. 372.

27. Ibid., p. 368.

28. Plato, *Dialogues, Cratylos,* as cited in Durant, *Life of Greece,* p. 371.

29. A. J. Toynbee, *Hellenism: The History of a Civilization* (New York: Oxford University Press, 1959), p. 95.

30. L. Minio-Paluello, "Aristotle," *Dictionary of Scientific Biography,* 1:250–81.

31. Durant, *Life of Greece,* p. 528; Minio-Paluello, "Aristotle," p. 279; M. Grant, *The Classical Greeks* (New York: Charles Scribner and Sons, 1989), pp. 250–68.

32. E. Clarke and J. Stannard, "Aristotle on the Anatomy of the Brain," *Journal of the History of Medicine and Allied Sciences* 18 (1963): 130–48; Von Staden, *Herophilus,* p. 157.

2. First Look into the Human Body, Third Century B.C.

1. P. M. Fraser, *Ptolemaic Alexandria* (Oxford: Clarendon Press, 1972).

2. E. A. Parsons, *The Alexandrian Library* (Amsterdam: Elsevier Press, 1952), p. 83.

3. Ibid., pp. 56, 71.

4. H. B. Gottschalk, "Strato of Lampsacus," *Dictionary of Scientific Biography* (New York: Charles Scribner and Sons, 1981), 13:91–95.

5. J. P. Mahaffy, *A History of Egypt Under the Ptolemaic Dynasty* (New York: Charles Scribner and Sons, 1899), p. 77; H. Von Staden, *Herophilus: The Art of Medicine in Early Alexandria* (New York: Cambridge University Press, 1989).

6. W. Durant, *Life of Greece,* vol. 2 of *Story of Civilization* (New York: Simon and Schuster, 1966), p. 590.

7. Fraser, *Ptolemaic Alexandria.*

8. J. A. Garraty and P. Gay, *The Columbia History of the World* (New York: Harper and Row, 1984), pp. 187–88.

9. C. G. Starr, *A History of the Ancient World* (New York: Oxford University Press, 1965), p. 415.

10. Parsons, *Alexandrian Library,* p. 211.

11. G. C. Pournaropoulos, "The Greek Medical School of Alexandria," *Proceedings from the XVII International Congress of the History of Medicine . . . 1960* (Athens and Kos: n.p., 1960), p. 314.

12. Fraser, *Ptolemaic Alexandria,* p. 330.

13. I. Asimov, "Aristarchus" in *Asimov's Biographical Encyclopedia of Science and Technology* (Garden City, N.Y.: Doubleday, 1972), p. 24.

14. J. Scarborough, "Celsus on Human Vivisection in Ptolemaic Alexandria," *Clio Medicine* 11 (1976): 25–38; G. B. Ferngren, "A Roman Declamation on Vivisection," *Transactions and Studies of the College of Physicians of Philadelphia* 5 (1982): 272–90; G. E. R. Lloyd, "Alcmaeon and the Early History of Dissection," *Sudhoffs Archiv* 59 (1975): 113–47.

15. Von Staden, *Herophilus,* p. 145.

16. J. Longrigg, "Herophilus," *Dictionary of Scientific Biography,* 6:317–19.

17. F. Solmsen, "Greek Philosophy and the Discovery of Nerves," *Museum Helveticum* 18 (1961): 150; J. Longrigg, "Praxagoras," *Dictionary of Scientific Biography,* 11:127.

18. Markellinos, *De Pulsibus,* as cited in C. R. S. Harris, *The Heart and Vascular System in Ancient Greek Medicine* (Oxford: Clarendon Press, 1973); Von Staden, *Herophilus,* pp. 282–84.

19. Pournaropoulos, "Greek Medical School," p. 311.

20. G. E. R. Lloyd, "A Note on Erasistratus of Ceos," *Journal of Hellenistic Studies* 95 (1975): 172; J. Longrigg, "Erasistratus," *Dictionary of Scientific Biography,* 4:382–86.

21. J. Longrigg, "Superlative Achievement and Comparative Neglect of Alexandrian Medical Science in Modern Historical Research," *History of Science* 19 (1981): 158.

22. Harris, *Heart and Vascular System,* p. 231; L. G. Wilson and F. Kudlien, "Galen," *Dictionary of Scientific Biography,* 5:227–37.

23. Harris, *Heart and Vascular System,* pp. 177–233.

24. Ibid., p. 196.

25. Ibid., p. 198.

26. Ibid., p. 195.

27. Ibid., p. 218.

28. Longrigg, "Erasistratus," pp. 382–86.

29. Caelius Aurelianus, *On Acute Diseases and on Chronic Diseases,* ed. and trans. I. E. Drabkin (Chicago: University of Chicago Press, 1950), pp. 753, 795.

30. Mahaffy, *History of Egypt,* p. 104.

31. E. P. Hoyt, *A Short History of Science: From the Middle Ages to the Present* (New York: John Day Company, 1966), p. 135; J. W. Estes, *The*

Medical Skills of Ancient Egypt (Canton, Mass.: Science History Publications, 1989), p. 32.

32. I. Asimov, "Eratosthenes," in *Asimov's Biographical Encyclopedia of Science and Technology* (Garden City, N.Y.: Doubleday and Company, 1972), p. 29.

33. Fraser, *Ptolemaic Alexandria,* p. 325.

34. T. Meyer-Steineg and K. Sudhoff, *Illustrierte Geschichte der Medizin,* 5th ed. (Stuttgart: G. Fischer, 1965), p. 61; W. H. F. Jones and T. L. Heath, "Medicine and Surgery," in *Cambridge Ancient History* (Cambridge, Eng.: Cambridge University Press, 1984), 7:321–52.

3. Years of Stagnation, 200 B.C.–A.D. 1450

1. J. P. Mahaffy, *A History of Egypt Under the Ptolemaic Dynasty* (New York: Charles Schuster and Sons, 1899), pp. 128–29; H. T. Davis, *Alexandria, the Golden City* (Evanston: Principia Press of Illinois, 1957), p. 139.

2. Polybius, *The Rise of the Roman Empire,* trans. I. Scott-Kilvert (London: Penguin, 1979), pp. 489–93.

3. W. H. F. Jones and T. L. Heath, "Hellenistic Science and Mathematics," in *Cambridge Ancient History* (Cambridge, Eng.: Cambridge University Press, 1984), 7:286.

4. Mahaffy, *History of Egypt,* p. 249.

5. Ibid., p. 124.

6. C. G. Starr, *A History of the Ancient World* (New York: Oxford University Press, 1965), p. 410.

7. Mahaffy, *History of Egypt,* pp. 163–66.

8. E. Guhl and W. Koner, *Everyday Life of the Greeks and Romans* (New York: Crescent Books, 1989).

9. Mahaffy, *History of Egypt,* p. 191.

10. P. M. Fraser, *Ptolemaic Alexandria* (Oxford: Clarendon Press, 1972).

11. F. Kudlien, "Rufus of Ephesus," *Dictionary of Scientific Biography* (New York: Charles Scribner and Sons, 1981), 11:602.

12. J. Bidez, *Alexandria,* in *Cambridge Ancient History* (Cambridge, Eng.: Cambridge University Press, 1965), 12:619–20.

13. L. G. Wilson and F. Kudlien, "Galen," *Dictionary of Scientific Biography,* 5:227–37.

14. T. Beck, "Galen," *Archiv für geschichte der Medizin* 3 (1909): 110–11.

15. Wilson and Kudlien, "Galen," p. 230.

16. A. Castiglioni, *A History of Medicine,* trans. E. B. Krumbhaar (New York: A. Knopf, 1958), p. 222.

17. J. M. Forrester, "An Experiment of Galen's Repeated," *Proceedings of the Royal Society of Medicine* 47 (1954): 242–43.

18. Wilson and Kudlien, "Galen," p. 235.

19. F. H. Garrison, *An Introduction to the History of Medicine* (Philadelphia: W. B. Saunders Company, 1961), p. 113; H. Saake, "Pneuma,"

Pauly-Wissowa's Realenzyclopädie der Klassischen Altertumswissenschaft, Supplement 14 (1972): 287–412.

20. Garrison, *History of Medicine,* p. 116.

21. S. N. Müller, *Caracalla,* vol. 12 of *Cambridge Ancient History* (Cambridge, Eng.: Cambridge University Press, 1965), p. 49.

22. Bidez, *Alexandria,* p. 619.

23. H. M. Gwatkin, "Christian Roman Empire and the Foundation of the Teutonic Kingdoms," *Cambridge Medieval History,* 8 vols. (Cambridge, Eng.: Cambridge University Press, 1911), 1:132.

24. *Encyclopedia Britannica,* 15th ed., s.v. "Theodosius."

25. W. Durant, *The Age of Faith,* vol. 4 of *Story of Civilization* (New York: Simon and Schuster, 1950), p. 282.

26. V. Sanford, *A Short History of Mathematics* (Boston: Houghton-Mifflin Co., 1958), p. 19; D. E. Smith, *History of Mathematics* (Boston: Ginn and Company, 1951–53), pp. 65–73.

27. A. N. Whitehead, *An Introduction to Mathematics* (New York: Oxford University Press, 1948), p. 43; G. Sarton, *Introduction to the History of Science* (Baltimore: Williams and Wilkins Company, 1948), p. 601; Sanford, *Short History of Mathematics,* p. 94.

28. Sanford, *Short History of Mathematics,* p. 95.

29. A. Hirsch, "Arabic Medicine," in *Biographisches Lexikon, Hervorragenden Aerzte* (Berlin: Urban and Schwarzenberg, 1927), pp. 165–66.

30. S. J. Haddad and A. Khairallah, "A Forgotten Chapter in the History of Blood Circulation," *Annotated Surgery* 104 (1936): 1; P. K. Hitti, *History of the Arabs from the Earliest Times to the Present* (New York: MacMillan, 1951); M. Meyerhof, "Al Kurashi Ibn Al Nafis," in *Enzyclopädie des Islam, Supplement* (Leiden: Brill, 1937).

31. J. L. Stipp, C. W. Hollister, and A. W. Dirrim, *The Rise and Development of Western Civilization* (New York: J. Wiley, 1974), p. 310.

32. Ibid., p. 290.

33. G. Roth, "Der schwarze Tod," *Ciba Symposium* 3 (1956): 195.

34. G. Boccaccio, *Decameron,* trans. J. M. Rigg (1921; reprint, New York: Dutton, 1973).

4. Renaissance: The Eye-Opener, 1450–1543

1. W. Durant, *The Age of Faith,* vol. 4 of *Story of Civilization* (New York: Simon and Schuster, 1950), pp. 714–21.

2. C. D. O'Malley, *Andreas Vesalius of Brussels, 1514–1564* (Berkeley: University of California Press, 1964).

3. Ibid., p. 15.

4. J. J. Norwich, *A History of Venice* (New York: A. Knopf, 1982), p. 274.

5. W. Durant, *The Renaissance,* vol. 5 of *Story of Civilization* (New York: Simon and Schuster, 1950), pp. 67–77.

6. G. Vasari, *Lives of the Most Eminent Painters, Sculptors and Architects,* trans. C. de Vere (New York: Crown Publishers, 1988).

7. Ibid.

8. Leonardo da Vinci, *I manoscritti di Leonardo da Vinci della Reale Biblioteca di Windsor: Dell'anatomia fogli B,* published by T. Sabachnikoff, transcribed and annotated by G. Piumanti (Turin: Roux and Viarengo, 1901), p. 21 (hereafter cited as *Fogli B*); E. MacCurdy, *The Notebooks of Leonardo da Vinci* (New York: Reynal and Hitchcock, 1938), pp. 103–288.

9. Leonardo da Vinci, *Quaderni d'Anatomia,* ed. and trans. O. C. L. Vangensten, A. Fonahn, and H. Hopstock (Christiania: J. Dybwad, 1911–16), 1:2–8 (hereafter cited as *Quaderni d'Anatomia*); K. D. Keele and C. Pedretti, *Leonardo da Vinci: Corpus of the Anatomical Studies in the Collection of Her Majesty the Queen at Windsor Castle* (London: Johnson Reprint Company, 1990), pp. 1978–80; C. D. O'Malley and J. B. de C. M. Saunders, *Leonardo da Vinci on the Human Body* (New York: Greenwich House, 1982).

10. W. von Seidlitz, *Leonardo da Vinci* (Vienna: Phaidon-Verlag, 1935).

11. R. Sabatini, *The Life of Cesare Borgia* (New York: Houghton Mifflin, 1924).

12. *Quaderni d'Anatomia,* 1:2–8.

13. Ibid., 1:13v.

14. Ibid., 1:12r; K. Clark and C. Pedretti, *A Catalogue of the Drawings of Leonardo da Vinci in the Collection of His Majesty the King, at Windsor Castle* (Cambridge, Eng.: Cambridge University Press, 1935).

15. *Quaderni d'Anatomia,* 3:8r.

16. *Fogli B,* p. 2v.

17. *Quaderni d'Anatomia,* 3:3v; R. H. Major, *A History of Medicine,* 2 vols. (Springfield, Ill.: Charles C Thomas, 1954), 1:377.

18. *Quaderni d'Anatomia,* 5:7r.

19. Ibid., 5:21r.

20. Leonardo da Vinci, *Il Codice Atlantico di Leonardo da Vinci nella Biblioteca Ambrosiana di Milano* (Milan: Hoepli, 1894–1904), p. 345v.

21. *Quaderni d'Anatomia,* 2:1r.

22. Ibid., 2:13v.

23. Leonardo da Vinci, *Codex Madrid* (New York: 1965), pp. 134v, 151v; C. Zamattio, *Mechanics of Water and Stone,* as cited in C. Zamattio, A. Marinoni, and A. M. Brizio, *Leonardo the Scientist* (New York: McGraw-Hill, 1980), p. 37.

24. *Quaderni d'Anatomia,* 2:12r; K. D. Keele, "Leonardo da Vinci's 'Anatomia Naturale,'" *Yale Journal of Biology and Medicine* 52 (1979): 369–409.

25. *Quaderni d'Anatomia,* 4:11v.

26. Keele and Pedretti, "Leonardo da Vinci," p. 376; F. Robicsek, "Leonardo da Vinci and the Sinuses of Valsalva," *Annals of Thoracic Surgery* 52 (1991): 328–35; *Quaderni d'Anatomia,* 2:13v.

27. H. Greenfield and W. Kolff, "The Prosthetic Heart Valve and Computer Graphics," *Journal of the American Medical Association* 219 (1972): 69; T. Doby, *Development of Angiography* (Littleton, Mass.:

Publishing Sciences Group, 1976), pp. 4–8.

28. *Fogli B,* p. 10v.

29. Ibid., p. 11v.

30. *Quaderni d'Anatomia,* 1:13v.

31. Leonardo da Vinci, *I manoscritti di Leonardo da Vinci della Reale Biblioteca di Windsor: Dell'anatomia fogli A,* published by T. Sabachnikoff, transcribed and annotated by G. Piumati (Paris: E. Rouveyre, 1898), p. 17.

32. Ibid., p. 8v; J. Wasserman, *Leonardo da Vinci* (New York: H. N. Abrams, 1975).

5. Results of a New Kind of Approach, 1543–1895

1. J. L. Stripp, C. W. Hollister, and A. W. Dirrim, *The Rise and Development of Western Civilization* (New York: Wiley, 1974), p. 488.

2. S. H. Steinberg, *Five Hundred Years of Printing* (New York: Penguin, 1977), p. 73.

3. M. Roth, ed., *Andreas Vesalius Bruxellensis* (1892; reprint, Amsterdam: Asher, 1965), p. 85.

4. C. D. O'Malley, *Andreas Vesalius of Brussels* (Berkeley: University of California Press, 1964), p. 113.

5. A. Vesalius, *Epistola re radicis chynae,* as cited in Roth, ed., *Andreas Vesalius Bruxellensis,* p. 139.

6. A. Vesalius, "De humani corporis fabrica," trans. B. Farrington, *Transactions of the Royal Society of South Africa* 20 (1931): 13.

7. C. D. O'Malley, "The Life and Times of Andreas Vesalius," *Annotated Western Medicine and Surgery* 5 (1951): 193.

8. O'Malley, *Andreas Vesalius,* p. 116.

9. E. Hintzsche, "Andreas Vesalius und sein Werk," *Ciba Zeitschrift* 9 (1946): 3655–62.

10. O'Malley, *Andreas Vesalius,* p. 177.

11. Ibid., preface.

12. Ibid.

13. F. H. Garrison, *An Introduction to the History of Medicine* (Philadelphia: Saunders, 1929), p. 220.

14. Hintzsche, "Andreas Vesalius," p. 3361.

15. J. Sylvius, *Vesani cuiusdem,* as cited in O'Malley, *Andreas Vesalius,* p. 250.

16. Ibid., p. 94.

17. Ibid., p. 126.

18. Ibid., preface.

19. A. Castiglioni, *A History of Medicine,* trans. E. B. Krumbhaar (New York: A. Knopf, 1958), p. 418.

20. Hintzsche, "Andreas Vesalius," p. 3362.

21. O'Malley, *Andreas Vesalius,* pp. 270–90.

22. A. Dide, *Michel Servet* (Vienna: n.p., 1925); H. Tollin, *Die Entdeckung des Blutkerislaufs durch Michel Servet (1511–1553)* (Jena: Dufft, 1876).

23. R. Colombo, *De re anatomica libri XV* (Venice: Berilacqua, 1559).

24. G. Falloppio, *Observationes anatomicae* (Venice: Apud Marcum Antonium Ulmum, 1561).

25. Hintzsche, "Andreas Vesalius," pp. 3663–73.

26. T. Doby, *Discoverers of Blood Circulation* (New York: Abelard-Schuman, 1963), p. 176.

27. O'Malley, *Andreas Vesalius,* p. 584.

28. O'Malley, "Life and Times of Andreas Vesalius," p. 197.

29. O'Malley, *Andreas Vesalius,* p. 309.

30. Hintzsche, "Andreas Vesalius," p. 3668.

31. J. J. Fahie, *Galileo, His Life and Work* (London: J. Murray, 1903), pp. 79–80.

32. R. S. Westfall, "Science and Patronage: Galileo and the Telescope," *Isis* 76 (1985): 11–30.

33. Fahie, *Galileo,* p. 208.

34. M. Rosenblum, "The History of the Microscope," *Proceedings of the Royal Microscopical Society* 2 (1967): 270.

35. J. Elmes, *Memoirs of the Life and Works of Sir Christopher Wren* (London: Priestly and Weale, 1823), p. 31.

36. R. Hooke, *Micrographia* (London: J. Martyn and J. Allestry, 1665); T. Doby, "Sir Christopher Wren and Medicine," *Episteme* 7 (1973): 83–106.

37. Castiglioni, *History of Medicine,* pp. 601–7.

38. S. Bradbury, *The Microscope: Past and Present* (New York: Pergamon Press, 1968), p. 134.

39. M. Klein, "J. M. Schleiden," *Dictionary of Scientific Biography* (New York: Charles Scribner and Sons, 1981), 11:174.

40. J. Steudel, "Johannes Müller," ibid., 9:572.

41. Rosenblum, "History of the Microscope," p. 285.

42. G. B. Risse, "Rudolf Virchow," *Dictionary of Scientific Biography,* 14:39–43; L. Clendening, *Source Book of Medical History* (New York: Dover, 1942), pp. 622–33.

43. Bradbury, *Microscope,* pp. 163–66.

44. Risse, "Rudolf Virchow," pp. 39–43.

45. Castiglioni, *History of Medicine,* pp. 729–35.

46. C. Bernard, *Cahier Rouge,* trans. H. H. Hoff and R. Guillemin (Cambridge, Mass.: Schenkman, 1967), p. 1.

47. P. Ehrlich, "Über die methylenblau reaction der lebenden Nervensubstanz," *Deutsche Medizinische Wochenschrift* 12 (1886): 49–52.

48. C. B. Holma, "Anticipating Changes in Neuroradiology," *American Journal of Roentgenology* 118 (1973): 701.

6. First Look into the Living Human Body, 1895–1913

1. R. McCorrmach, "Hertz," *Dictionary of Scientific Biography* (New York: Charles Scribner and Sons, 1981), 6:348.

2. "Plucker and Hittorf," *Radiography and Clinical Photography* 5 (1931): 1.

3. M. Brucer, *Vignettes in Nuclear Medicine,* no. 93 (St. Louis: Mallinckrodt Chemical Works, 1978), p. 9.

4. W. Crookes, "Radiant Matter," as cited in W. H. Brock, "William Crookes," *Dictionary of Scientific Biography,* 3–4:474–82.

5. O. Glasser, *Dr. W. C. Röntgen,* 2d ed. (Springfield, Ill.: Charles C Thomas, 1958), p. 85.

6. I. Asimov, "Kelvin" and "W. Thomson," in *Asimov's Encyclopedia of Science and Technology* (Garden City, N.Y.: Doubleday, 1972), p. 379.

7. Glasser, *Dr. W. C. Röntgen,* p. 40.

8. Asimov, "Hertz," *Asimov's Encyclopedia,* p. 715.

9. Ibid.

10. A. L. Herman, "Philip Lenard," *Dictionary of Scientific Biography,* 10:181.

11. Glasser, *Dr. W. C. Röntgen,* p. 23.

12. Ibid., p. 36.

13. Ibid., p. 39.

14. W. C. Röntgen, *Über Eine neue Art von Strahlen* (Würzurg: Stahel, 1895).

15. Ibid.

16. Ibid.

17. E. A. Codman, "Letter Written in 1901," in *Classic Descriptions in Diagnostic Roentgenology,* ed. A. J. Bruwer, 2 vols. (Springfield, Ill.: Charles C Thomas, 1964), 1:324 (hereafter cited as *Classic Descriptions*).

18. H. J. W. Dam, "Interview with Roentgen," as cited in P. Donizetti, *Shadow and Substance* (Oxford: Pergamon Press, 1967), pp. 35–39.

19. E. R. N. Grigg, *The Trail of the Invisible Light* (Springfield, Ill.: Charles C Thomas, 1965), p. 836.

20. *Classic Descriptions,* 1:57; H. C. Thurstan, "X Rays in 1896," *Liverpool Medico-Chirurgical Journal* 45 (1937): 61–77.

21. H. R. Schinz, *Sechzig Jahre Medzinische Radiologie* (Stuttgart: G. Thieme, 1959), pp. 109–16.

22. *Classic Descriptions,* 1:345–65.

23. Ibid., pp. 399–407.

24. J. MacIntyre, "Roentgen Rays: Photography of Renal Calculus," *Lancet* 2 (1896): 118.

25. T. Tuffier, as cited in S. E. Duplay and P. Reclus, *Traité de Chirurgie* (Paris: Masson, 1897–1899), 7:412.

26. G. Illyés, "Ureter catheterezés és radiographia," *Orvosi Hetilap* 45 (1901): 659–62.

27. F. Voelker and A. von Lichtenberg, "Pyelographie," *Münchener Medizinische Wochenschrift* 53 (1906): 105.

28. A. von Lichtenberg and H. Dietlen, "Darstellung des Nierenbeckens und Ureters nach Sauerstoff-füllung," *Münchener Medizinische Wochenschrift* 58 (1911): 1341.

29. W. T. Belfield, "Skiagraphy of the seminal ducts," *Journal of the American Medical Association* 60 (1913): 800.

30. O. Riethus, "Über einen Fall von Schussverletzung des Herzens," *Deutsche Zeitschrift für Chirurgie* 67 (1903): 416–46; G. Hoppe-Seyler, "Über die Verwendung der Röntgenstrahlen zur Diagnose der Arteriosklerose," *Münchener Medizinische Wochenschrift* 13 (1896): 316.

31. E. Haschek and T. O. Lindenthal, "Ein Beitrag zur praktischen Verwertung der Photographie nach Röntgen," *Wiener Klinische Wochenschrift* 9 (1896): 63.

32. Schinz, *Sechzig Jahre Medzinische Radiologie*, p. 152.

33. Grigg, *Trail of Invisible Light*, p. 193.

34. B. Sabat, "A Radiographic Method of Recording Movements of the Diaphragm, Heart and Aorta," *Lwowsky Tygodn. Lekar.* 6 (1911): 395.

35. F. Trendelenburg, "Projectile in Heart," as cited in O. Franck and W. Alwens, "Kreislaufstudien am Röntgenschirm," *Münchener Medizinische Wochenschrift* 57 (1910): 950–54; A. Podres, "Projectile in Heart," *Fortschritte der Chirurgie* (1898): 512.

36. R. Haecker, "Experimentelle Studien zur Pathologie und Chirurgie des Herzens," *Archiv für Klinische Chirurgie* 84 (1907): 1035–98.

37. Revensdorf, "Darstellung Experimenteller Luftembolie in Röntgenogramm," *Fortschritte auf dem Gebiete der Röntgenstrahlen* 12 (1908): 22–24 (hereafter cited as *Fortschritte Röntgenstrahlen*).

38. Franck and Alwens, "Kreislaufstudien am Röntgenschirm."

39. W. Alwens and W. Frick, "Über die Lokalisation von Luftembolien in der Lunge," *Frankfurter Zeitschrift für Pathologie* 15 (1914): 315–26.

40. T. Doby, *Development of Angiography* (Littleton, Mass.: Publishing Sciences Group, 1976), p. 43.

41. *Classic Descriptions,* 2:1774–96.

42. W. B. Cannon, "The Movements of the Stomach Studied by Means of the Roentgen Rays," *American Journal of Physiology* 1 (1898): 359–82.

43. A. C. Barger, "New Technology for a New Century: W. B. Cannon and the Invisible Rays," *American Journal of Roentgenology* 136 (1981): 187–95.

44. F. H. Williams, *The Roentgen Ray in Medicine and Surgery* (New York: MacMillan Company, 1901).

45. J. Ch. Roux and Balthasard, "Études des contractions de l'estomac chez l'homme à l'aide des rayons de Roentgen," *Comptes Rendus de Séances de la Société de Biologie et des ses Filiales* 10 (1897): 785.

46. H. Rieder, "Radiologische Untersuchungen des Magens und Darms beim lebenden Menschen," *Münchener Medizinische Wochenschrift* 51 (1904): 1548.

47. C. Kestle, H. Rieder, and J. Rosenthal, "Über kinematographisch aufgenommene Röntgenogramme," *Münchener Medizinische Wochenschrift* 56 (1909): 280.

48. C. Bachem and H. Guenther, "Bariumsulfat als schattenbildendes Kontrastmittel bei Röntgenuntersuchungen," *Zeitschrift für Röntgenkunde und Radiumforschung* 12 (1910): 369.

49. J. von Elischer, "Über eine Methode zur Röntgenuntersuchung des Magens," *Fortschritte Röntgenstrahlen* 18 (1911): 332–40.

50. G. Forsell, "Über die Beziehung der Röntgenbilder des menschlichen Magens zu seinem Bau," *Fortschritte Röntgenstrahlen* 30 (1913): 137.

51. Schuele, "Über die Sondierung und Radiographie des Dickdarmes," *Archiv für Verdauungs-Krankheiten* 10 (1904): 11–118.

52. F. Haenisch, "Die Röntgenuntersuchung bei Verengungen des Dickdarms," *Münchener Medizinische Wochenschrift* 70 (1923): 2375.

53. Robinsohn and Werndorff, "Eine neue Methode in der Diagnostick der Gelenkerkrankungen," *Zentralblatt für Chirurgie* 2 (1905): 826.

54. A. Lorey, "Demonstration einiger seltener Röntgenbefunde," *Verhandlungen der Deutschen Rtg. Gesellschaft* 8 (1912): 52.

55. A. Feldman, "A Sketch of the Technical History of Radiology from 1896 to 1920," *Radio-Graphics* 9 (1989): 1113–28.

56. A. W. Fuchs, *On Aperture Diaphragms and Cones,* as cited in *Classic Descriptions,* 1:124.

57. R. Brecher and E. Brecher, *The Rays: A History of Radiology in the U.S. and Canada* (Baltimore: Williams and Wilkins Company, 1969), p. 52.

58. H. C. Snook, "A New Roentgen Generator," *Archives of the Roentgen Ray* 13 (1908): 186–88.

59. O. Pasche, "Über eine neue Blendenvorrichtung in der Röntgentechnik," *Deutsche Medizinische Wochenschrift* 1 (1903): 266.

60. G. Bucky, "Über die Ausschaltung der . . . Sekunderstrahlen," *Verhandlungen der Deutschen Rtg. Gesellschaft* 9 (1913): 30–32.

61. H. E. Potter, "Diaphragming Roentgen Rays," *American Journal of Roentgenology* 3 (1916): 142–45; W. M. Angus, "A Commentary in the Development of Diagnostic Imaging Technology," *Radio-Graphics* 9 (1989): 1225–44; N. Knight, "Seventy-Five Years of RSNA Approaching a Century of Radiology," *Radio-Graphics* 9 (1989): 1101–12.

7. Technical Advances, Contrast Materials, and Radioactivity, 1913–1944

1. R. Brecher and E. Brecher, *The Rays: A History of Radiology in the United States and Canada* (Baltimore: Williams and Wilkins Company, 1969), p. 192.

2. E. D. Trout, "Tubes and Generators," in *Classic Descriptions of Diagnostic Roentgenology,* ed. A. J. Bruwer, 2 vols. (Springfield, Ill.: Charles C Thomas, 1964), 1:213–23 (hereafter cited as *Classic Descriptions*).

3. W. D. Coolidge, "Vacuum Tube," Application to the United States Patent Office, May 13, 1913.

4. Brecher and Brecher, *Rays,* p. 197.

5. S. B. Dewing, *Modern Radiology in Historical Perspective* (Springfield, Ill.: Charles C Thomas, 1962), p. 75.

6. A. W. Fuchs and G. N. Corney, *Radiographic Recording Media* (Springfield, Ill.: Charles C Thomas, 1965), pp. 97–119.

7. A. W. Fischer, "Über eine neue Röntgenologische Untersuchungsmethode des Dickdarmes," *Klinische Wochenschrift* 2 (1923): 1595–98.

8. G. Heuer and W. E. Dandy, "Roentgenography in the Localization of Brain Tumor," *Johns Hopkins Bulletin* 27 (1916): 331.

9. W. E. Dandy, "Ventriculography Following the Injection of Air into the Cerebral Ventricles," *Annotated Surgery* 68 (1918): 5–11.

10. J. W. D. Bull, "History of Neuroradiology," *British Journal of Radiology* 34 (1961): 69–84.

11. Mourier, "In Memoriam: J. A. Sicard," *Marseilles Médicine* 67 (1930): 331.

12. J. Forestier, "Sicard et son œvre radiologique," *La Médicine* 10 (1970): 466–70.

13. B. S. Epstein, "Myelography," in *Classic Descriptions,* 1:941–65.

14. J. A. Sicard and J. Forestier, *The Use of Lipiodol in Diagnosis and Treatment: A Clinical and Radiological Survey* (London: Oxford University Press, H. Milford, 1932).

15. Ibid.

16. J. A. Sicard and J. Forestier, "Injections Intravasculaires d'huile iodée sous contrôl radiologique," *Comptes Rendus de Séances de la Société de Biologie et des ses Filiales* 88 (1923): 1200.

17. W. H. Cole, "Historical Features of Cholecyctography," *Radiology* 76 (1961): 354–75.

18. E. A. Graham and W. H. Cole, "Roentgenologic Examination of the Gall Bladder," *Journal of the American Medical Association* 82 (1924): 613–14.

19. C. A. Waters, S. Bayne-Jones, and L. G. Rowntree, "Roentgenography of the Lungs: Roentgenographic Studies in Living Animals after Intratracheal Injection of Iodoform Emulsion," *Archives of Internal Medicine* 19 (1917): 538–49.

20. E. D. Osborne et al., "Roentgenography of Urinary Tract During Excretion of Sodium Iodide," *Journal of the American Medical Association* 80 (1923): 368–73.

21. T. Doby, *Development of Angiography* (Littleton, Mass.: Publishing Sciences Group, 1976), pp. 58–63.

22. J. Berberich and S. Hirsch, "Röntgenographische Darstellung der Arterien und Venen am Iebenden Menschen," *Klinische Wochenschrift* 2 (1923): 226–28.

23. B. Brooks, "Intraarterial Injection of Sodium Iodide," *Journal of the American Medical Association* 82 (1924): 1016–19.

24. B. Brooks and F. A. Jostes, "A Clinical Study of Diseases of the Circulation of Extremities," *Archives of Surgery* 9 (1924): 485–503.

25. E. Moniz, *Confidencias de um investigador cientifico* (Lisbon: Atica, 1949).

26. Ibid.

27. E. Moniz, *Diagnostic des tumeurs cérébrales et épreuve de l'encéphalographie artérielle* (Paris: Masson et cie, 1931).

28. Moniz, *Confidencias.*

29. R. Dos Santos, A. C. Lamas, and J. P. Caldas, *Artériographie des membres de l'aorte abdominale* (Paris: Masson et cie, 1931).

30. M. Swick, "Darstellung der Niere und Harnwege," *Klinische Wochenschrift* 8 (1929): 2087–89.

31. W. Forssmann, "Die Sondierung des rechten Herzens," *Klinische Wochenschrift* 8 (1929): 2085–87.

32. Forssmann, *Selbstversuch, Erinnerungen eines Chirurgen* (Düsseldorf: Droste, 1972).

33. Forssmann, personal communication to T. Doby, 1969.

34. Forssmann, "Über Kontrastdarstellung der Höhlen des lebenden Herzens und der Lungenschlagader," *Münchener Medizinische Wochenschrift* 78 (1931): 490–92.

35. Doby, *Development of Angiography,* p. 129.

36. R. J. Reynolds, "Cinematography," *American Journal of Roentgenology* 33 (1935): 522–28.

37. J. D. Bricker, "Tomography," in *Classic Descriptions,* 2:1406–12.

38. A. Vallebona, "Una modalità di technica per la dissociazione radiografica," *Radiologia Medica* 17 (1930): 1090–97.

39. Z. des Plantes, "Een bijzondere methode . . . , " *Nederlanch Tijdschrift voor Geneeskunde* 75 (1931): 5218–22; G. Grossmann, "Tomographie," *Fortschritte Röntgenstrahlen* 51 (1935): 61–80, 191–208.

40. "Béla Alexander," *Medicor News* 1 (1974): 11.

41. Z. des Plantes, "Subtraction," *Fortschritte Röntgenstrahlen* 52 (1935): 69.

42. A. Castellanos, R. Pereiras, and A. Garcia, "La angio-cardiografia radio-opaqua," *Archivos de la Sociedad de Estudios Clinicos de la Habaña* 31 (1937): 223–96.

43. G. P. Robb and I. Steinberg, "Visualization of the Chambers of the Heart: The Pulmonary Circulation and the Great Blood Vessels in Man, a Practical Method," *American Journal of Roentgenology* 41 (1939): 1–17.

44. I. Steinberg, personal communication to T. Doby, 1965.

45. M. Oka, "Eine neue Methode zur Röntgenologischen Darstellung der Milz," *Fortschritte Röntgenstrahlen* 40 (1929): 497–501; P. Radt, "Eine Methode zur Röntgenologischen Kontrastdarstellung von Milz und Leber," *Klinische Wochenschrift* 8 (1929): 2128–29.

46. G. von Hevesy and F. Paneth, "RaD als 'Indikator' des Bleies," *Zeitschrift für Anorganische Chemie* 82 (1913): 322.

47. G. von Hevesy, "The Absorption of and Translocation of Lead by Plants," *Biochemistry Journal* 17 (1923): 439.

48. G. von Hevesy, "Über Anwendung von radioactiven Indika toren in der Biologie," *Biochemische Zeitschrift* 173 (1926): 175.

49. C. Schmidt, "George de Hevesy, Nuclear Medicine Pioneer," *Applied Radiology* 6 (1977): 56.

50. A. S. Freedberg, "In Memoriam: Herman L. Blumgart," *Journal of Nuclear Medicine* 19 (1978): 569.

51. F. Joliot and I. Curie, "Artificial Production of a New Kind of Radioelement," *Nature* 133 (1934): 201.

52. E. Fermi, "Radioactivity Induced by Neutron Bombardment," *Nature* 133 (1934): 757.

53. H. Levi, "George de Hevesy," *Nuclear Physics* 98 (1967): 1; O. Chievitz and G. von Hevesy, "Radioactive Indicator in the Study of Phosphorus Metabolism in Rats," *Nature* 136 (1935): 754.

54. L. Hahn and G. von Hevesy, "A Method of Blood Volume Determination," *Acta Physiologica Scandinavica* 1 (1940): 3.

55. L. Hahn and G. von Hevesy, "Turnover Rate of Nucleic Acid," *Nature* 145 (1940): 549; L. Hahn, G. von Hevesy, and W. D. Armstrong, "Exchange of Radiophosphorus by Dentine Enamel," *Journal of Biology and Chemistry* 133 (1940): 14.

56. M. Brucer, *Vignettes of Nuclear Medicine,* no. 90 (St. Louis: Mallinckrodt Chemical Works, 1979), p. 1.

57. J. G. Hamilton, "Rates of Absorption of Radio-Sodium in Normal Human Subjects," *Proceedings of the National Academy of Science* 23 (1937): 521.

58. W. L. Laurence, *Men and Atoms* (New York: Simon and Schuster, 1962).

8. More Technology Helps to See More: 1940s, 1950s, and 1960s

1. R. H. Morgan, "Photoelectric Timing Mechanism for Automatic Control of Roentgenographic Exposure," *American Journal of Roentgenology* 48 (1942): 220–28.

2. E. R. N. Grigg, *The Trail of the Invisible Light* (Springfield, Ill.: Charles C Thomas, 1965), p. 434.

3. Ibid., p. 418.

4. G. Amheuille et al., "Remarques sur quelques cas d'artériographie pulmonaire chez l'homme vivant," *Bulletins et Mémoires de la Société de Médecine de Paris* 60 (1935): 729.

5. A. Cournand, "Cardiac Catheterization," *Acta Medica Scandinavica,* Supp. 579 (1975).

6. Ibid.

7. P. L. Fariñas, "A New Technique for the Arteriographic Examination of the Abdominal Aorta and Its Branches," *American Journal of Roentgenology* 46 (1941): 641–45; S. Radner, "Thoracal Aortography by Catheterization," *Acta Radiologica Scandinavica* 29 (1948): 179–80.

8. E. C. Peirce, "Percutaneous Femoral Artery Catheterization in Man with Special Reference to Aortography," *Surgery, Gynecology and Obstetrics* 93 (1951): 56–74.

9. E. H. Euler, "Die Peroesophageale Aortenpunktion," *Archiv für Ohren-, Nasen- und Kehlkopfheilkunde* 155 (1949): 536–67.

10. E. R. Ponsdomenech and V. Beato-Nuñez, "Heart Puncture in Man for Diodrast Visualization of the Ventricular Chambers and Great Arteries," *American Heart Journal* 41 (1951): 643–50.

11. I. Chavez, "Thirty Years' Progress in Cardiological Diagnosis," *American Journal of Cardiology* 1 (1958): 3–18.

12. G. Jönsson, "Thoracic Aortography by Means of a Cannula," *Acta Radiologica Scandinavica* 31 (1949): 376–86.

13. S. I. Seldinger, personal letter to T. Doby, 1976.

14. Seldinger, "Catheter Replacement of the Needle in Percutaneous Arteriography (A New Technique)," *Acta Radiologica Scandinavica* 39 (1953): 368–76.

15. F. M. Sones and E. K. Shirey, "Ciné Coronary Arteriography," *Modern Concepts of Cardiovascular Disease* 31 (1962): 735; P. Ödman, "Percutaneous Selective Angiography of the Main Branches of the Aorta," *Acta Radiologica Scandinavica* 45 (1956): 1–14; T. Doby, "A Tribute to Sven Ivar Seldinger," *American Journal of Roentgenology* 142 (1984): 1–3.

16. Nobelstiftelsen, *Nobel Lectures, Including Presentation Speeches and Laureates' Biographies,* vol. 3 (Amsterdam: Elsevier Publishing Company, 1964), p. 499.

17. M. Brucer, *Vignettes of Nuclear Medicine,* no. 90 (1978), p. 8.

18. M. Brucer, "Nuclear Medicine Begins with a Boa Constrictor," *Journal of Nuclear Medicine* 19 (1978): 595.

19. G. J. Hine, "The Inception of Photoelectric Scintillation Detection," *Journal of Nuclear Medicine* 18 (1977): 868.

20. M. Deutsch, "Naphthalene Counters for Beta and Gamma Rays," *Nucleonics* 2 (1948): 58.

21. R. Hofstadter, "Alkali Halide Scintillation Counters," *Physiological Reviews* 74 (1948): 100.

22. B. Cassen, L. Curtis, C. Reed, and R. Libby, "Instrumentation for [131]I Use in Medical Studies," *Nucleonics* 9 (1951): 46.

23. H. O. Anger, "Scintillation Camera," *Review of Scientific Instruments* 29 (1958): 159.

24. H. O. Anger, "Tomography and Other Depth-Discrimination Techniques," *Instruments in Nuclear Medicine* 2 (1974): 62.

25. H. Wagner, "Images of the Future," *Journal of Nuclear Medicine* 19 (1978): 599.

26. G. E. Donovan, "Radiology in Color," *Lancet* 1:15 (April 14, 1951): 832–33.

27. J. L. Bonnan, "Color Roentgenography," in *Classic Descriptions in Diagnostic Roentgenology,* ed. A. J. Bruwer, 2 vols. (Springfield, Ill.: Charles C Thomas, 1964), 2:1120–23 (hereafter cited as *Classic Descriptions*).

28. R. Schindler, "Ein Völlig ungefährliches flexibles Gastroskop," *Münchener Medizinische Wochenschrift* 79 (1932): 1268.

29. A. C. S. Van Heel, "A New Method of Transporting Optical Images Without Aberration," *Nature* 173 (1954): 39.

30. J. L. Baird, British Patent Special Number 20, 969/27-1929.

31. H. H. Hopkins and N. S. Kapany, "A Flexible Fiberscope Using Static Scanning," *Nature* 173 (1954): 39.

32. B. J. Hirschowitz, "A Personal History of the Fiberscope," *Gastroenterology* 76 (1979): 864–69.

33. P. R. Salmon, *Fiber-optic Endoscopy* (New York: Grune and Stratton, 1974), p. 237.

34. B. J. Hirschowitz, L. E. Curtiss, C. W. Peters, and H. M. Pollard, "Demonstration of a New Gastroscope, the Fiberscope," *Gastroenterology* 35 (1958): 50.

35. S. Tasaka and S. Ashizawa, "Studies on Gastric Diseases Using the Gastrocamera," *American Gastroscopic Society* (1958): 12.

36. W. I. Wolff and H. Shinya, "Modern Endoscopy of the Alimentary Tract," *Current Problems in Surgery* 8 (1974): 1–62.

37. T. R. Liebermann and M. Barnes, "Gastrointestinal Fiberoptic Endoscopy," *Surgical Clinics of North America* 59 (1979): 794; W. I. Wolff, M. B. Grossmann, et al., "Angiodysplasia of the Colon, Diagnosis and Treatment," *Gastroenterology* 72 (1977): 329.

38. G. Rizk, R. Goodale, and K. Amplatz, "Vascular Endoscopy," *Radiology* 106 (1973): 33–35; J. F. Vollmar and L. W. Storz, "Vascular Endoscopy," *Surgical Clinics of North America* 54 (1974): 111–22.

39. S. Bradbury, *The Microscope: Past and Present* (Oxford: Pergamon Press, 1968), p. 212.

40. Ibid., p. 228.

41. P. Goby, "X Ray Magnifications," *Comptes Rendus de l'Academie des Sciences* 156 (1913): 686.

42. C. P. Oderr, "X Ray Microscopy," in *Classic Descriptions,* 2:1067.

43. A. A. Barklay, "Microarteriography," *British Journal of Radiology* 20 (1942): 394–404.

44. S. V. Grechishkin and M. G. Prives, "Weiche Röntgenstrahlen in Medizin und Embryologie," *Vesn. Rentg. Radiology* 14 (1935): 14.

45. P. Rubin et al., "Microangiography as a Technique," *American Journal of Roentgenology* 92 (1964): 378–87.

46. A. Vallebona, "Studio di un metodo di microradiografia," *Liguria Medica* 13 (1928).

47. C. A. Beam, "Macroradiography," in *Classic Descriptions,* 2:1021–23.

48. G. J. Van der Plaats, "Prinzipien, Technik und medizinische Anwendung der radiologishen Vergrösserungstechnik," *Fortschritte Röntgenstrahlen* 77 (1952): 605–10; K. Komiyama, "Size of the Focal Spot on Auto-Bias X Ray Tube," *Nippon Acta Radiologica* 14 (1954): 487–94.

49. S. Takahashi and S. Sakuma, *Magnification Radiography* (New York: Springer-Verlag, 1975).

50. J. M. Bramble and A. W. Templeton, "The Importance of

Magnification Radiology in the Modern Diagnostic Imaging Department," *Electromedica* 55 (1987): 91.

51. A. Salomon, "Beiträge zur Pathologie und Klinik der Mammakarzinome," *Archiv für Klinische Chirurgie* 101 (1913): 573–668.

52. S. L. Warren, "A Roentgenologic Study of the Breast," *American Journal of Roentgenology* 24 (1930): 113–24.

53. R. Leborgne, C. M. Dominguez, and J. A. Mautone, "Diagnostico de los tumores de la mama," *Boletin de la Sociedad Cirurgia Uruguay* 20 (1949): 407–22.

54. L. Egan, "Experience with Mammography in a Tumor Institution," *Radiology* 75 (1960): 894–900.

55. C. M. Gros, "Méthodologie, Symposium sur la sein," *Journal de Radiologie et d'Electrologie* 48 (1967): 638–55.

56. H. R. Gould et al., "Xeroradiography of the Breast," *American Journal of Roentgenology* 84 (1960): 220–23.

57. M. Curie, *Pierre Curie,* trans. C. and V. Kellogg (New York: Dover Publishers Incorporated, 1963), p. 21.

58. C. Schueler, H. Lee, and G. Wade, "Fundamentals of Digital Ultrasonic Imaging," *IEEE Transactions on Sonics and Ultrasonics* 31 (1984): 195.

59. J. Thurzò, *Craniotonoscopy According to Benedek* (Debrecen, Hung.: Debrecen University, 1932), 227.

60. K. T. Dussik, "Über die Moeglichkeit hochfrequente Mechanische Schwingungen als diagnostisches Hilfsmittel zu verwenden," *Zeitschrift für die Gesamte Neurologie und Psychiatrie* 174 (1942): 153.

61. D. L. King, *Diagnostic Ultrasound* (St. Louis: Mosby, 1974), p. 4.

62. D. E. Howry and W. R. Bliss, "Ultrasonic Visualization of Soft Tissue Structures of the Body," *Journal of Laboratory Clinical Medicine* 40 (1952): 579; King, *Diagnostic Ultrasound,* p. 4.

63. I. Edler and C. H. Gertz, "The Use of Ultrasonic Reflectoscope for the Continuous Recording of the Movements of Heart Walls," *K. Fysiogr. Saellsk. Lund Foerh.* 24 (1954): 1.

64. S. Satomura, "Ultrasonic Doppler Method for the Inspection of Cardiac Functions," *Journal of the Acoustical Society of America* 29 (1957): 1181.

65. L. Leksell, "Echoencephalography: Detection of Intracranial Complications Following Head Injury," *Acta Chirurgica Scandinavica* 110 (1955): 301.

66. G. H. Mundt and W. F. Hughes, "Ultrasonics in Ocular Diagnosis," *American Journal of Ophthalmology* 41 (1956): 488; I. Donald, J. MacVicar, and T. G. Brown, "Investigation of Abdominal Masses by Pulsed Ultrasound," *Lancet* 1 (June 7, 1958): 1188.

67. M. Viikeri, "Ultrasound Examination of Pleural Plaques," *Acta Radiologica Scandinavica Supplement* 301 (1970): 12.

68. K. J. W. Taylor, *Atlas of Gray Scale Ultrasonography* (New York: Churchill Livingstone, 1978), p. 8.

69. J. B. Kinmonth, G. W. Taylor, and R. K. Harper, "Lymph-angiography: A Technique for Its Clinical Use in the Lower Limb," *British Medical Journal* 1 (1955): 940–42.

70. S. Wallace et al., "Lymphangiograms: Their Diagnostic and Therapeutic Potential," *Radiology* 76 (1961): 179–99.

9. A Great Leap from Tiny Chips: Computerization, 1960s and 1970s

1. W. R. Handee, "Cross Sectional Medical Imaging," *Radio-Graphics* 9 (1989): 1155–80.

2. B. J. M., "CT Scanning Recognized with Nobel Prize," *Journal of the American Medical Association* 242 (1979): 2380; "Allan MacLeod Cormack," in *Encyclopedia of Nobel Prize Winners,* ed. F. Veszits (Budapest: Gondolat Publishing Company, 1985).

3. H. H. Goldstein, *The Computer from Pascal to Von Neumann* (Princeton: Princeton University Press, 1972); M. L. Dertouzos and J. Moses, eds., *The Computer Age: A Twenty-Year View* (Cambridge, Mass.: MIT Press, 1983), p. 242.

4. R. Moreau, *The Computer Comes of Age,* trans. J. Hawlett (Cambridge, Mass.: MIT Press, 1984), p. 134.

5. Giscard d'Estaing, "Letter Written to S. Nora," in S. Nora and A. Minc, *The Computerization of Society: A Report to the President of France* (Cambridge, Mass.: MIT Press, 1980), p. 17.

6. T. D. Sterling, J. Nickson, and S. V. Pollack, "Is Medical Diagnosis a General Computer Problem?" *Journal of the American Medical Association* 198 (1966): 191; R. Paycha, "Aide en diagnostic des affections retiniennes," *Presse Médicale* 65 (1957): 26–28.

7. M. S. Potsaid et al., "Computer Analysis of Radiographs," *Medical Sciences* (March 1966): 35.

8. R. Kumar and S. N. Srihari, "An Expert System for the Interpretation of Cranial CT Scan Images," *IEEE Transactions on Sonics and Ultrasonics* 32 (1985): 548–55.

9. "Godfrey Hounsfield," in *Current Biography* (New York: H. W. Wilson Company, 1980), 153–55.

10. Ibid.

11. G. N. Hounsfield, "Computed Tomography," in *Medical Imaging: CT, NMR,* ed. L. Kreel and R. E. Steiner (Aylesbury, Eng.: H. M. and M. Publishing, 1979), pp. 1–9.

12. J. Bull, *History of Computed Tomography in Radiology of the Skull and Brain,* ed. T. H. Newton and G. D. Potts (St. Louis: C. V. Mosby Company, 1981), pp. 3835–49.

13. J. Scatliff, personal communication to T. Doby, 1973.

14. Hounsfield, "Computed Tomography," pp. 1–9.

15. Ibid.

16. J. Ambrose and G. Hounsfield, "Computerized Transverse Axial Tomography," *British Journal of Radiology* 46 (1973): 148–49.

17. Correspondence with Scatliff; see also Bull, *History of Computed Tomography,* pp. 3835–49.

18. P. F. J. New et al., "Computerized Tomography with the EMI Scanner," *Radiology* 110 (1974): 109–23; P. F. J. New and W. R. Scott, *Computed Tomography of the Brain and Orbit* (Baltimore: Williams and Wilkins Company, 1975); L. Menzer, T. Sabin, and V. H. Mark, "Computerized Axial Tomography: Use in the Diagnosis of Dementia," *Journal of the American Medical Association* 234 (1975): 754–57.

19. G. M. McCulloch and K. Lille, *CT Scanners: A Technical Report* (Chicago: American Hospital Association, 1977); G. Alker, S. Rudin, and D. Bednarek, "Computed Tomography," in *Encyclopedia of Medical Devices and Instrumentation,* ed. J. G. Webster (New York: John Wiley and Sons, 1988).

20. R. S. Ledley, "Innovation and Creativeness in Scientific Research: A Personal Experience in the Development of Computerized Axial Tomography" and "Editorial," *Computers in Biology and Medicine* 4 (1974): 133–36; R. S. Ledley et al., "Computerized X Ray Tomography of the Human Body," *Science* 186 (1974): 207–12; "Scanner Gives Colorful View of Patients," *Journal of the American Medical Association* 229 (1974): 1025–26; D. Schellinger et al., "Early Clinical Experience with the ACTA Scanner," *Radiology* 114 (1975): 257–61.

21. F. E. Glasauer and G. Alker, "Metrizamide Enhanced Computed Tomography: An Adjunct to Myelography in Lumbar Disc Herniation," *Computer Radiology* 5 (1983): 305–10.

22. G. Alker, "Demonstration of Fractured Teeth by CT Scanning," unpublished manuscript, 1987, Alker family, Williamsville, N.Y.

23. G. Kossoff, "Improved Techniques in Ultrasonic Cross Sectional Echography," *Ultrasonics* 10 (1972): 222–27.

24. G. Kossoff et al., "Principles and Classification of Soft Tissues by Gray Scale Echography," *Ultrasonics in Medicine and Biology* 2 (1976): 89–105.

25. S. Satomura et al., "Memoirs of the Institute of Scientific and Industrial Research," *Osaka University Annals* 13 (1955): 125.

26. D. W. Baker, S. A. Rubenstein, and G. S. Lorch, "Pulsed Doppler Echocardiography," *American Journal of Medicine* 63 (1977): 69.

27. D. W. Baker, "Application of Pulsed Doppler Techniques," *Radiological Clinics of North America* 18 (1980).

28. R. Omoto et al., *Color Atlas of Real Time Dimensional Doppler Echocardiography* (Tokyo: Shindan-To-Chiryo, 1984).

29. W. M. Blackhear et al., "Detection of Carotid Occlusive Disease by Ultrasound Imaging and Pulsed Doppler Spectrum Analysis," *Surgery* 86 (1979): 698–706; D. H. Leary and J. F. Polak, "Interrogating the Carotid with Color Doppler Imaging," *Diagnostic Imaging* (1988): 204–10.

30. L. S. Graham, J. G. Kereiakes, C. Harris, and M. B. Cohen, "Nuclear Medicine from Becquerel to the Present," *Radio-Graphics* 9 (1989): 1189–1202.

31. G. Finlayson, "PET and Overview," *Applied Radiology* 18 (1989): 10–14.

32. B. L. Holman, T. C. Hill, and J. L. Moretti, *SPECT Brain Imaging with Iofetamine in Stroke: A Clinical Update* (Milwaukee: Medical College of Wisconsin, 1988).

33. B. L. Holman and S. S. Tumeh, "Single Photon Emission Tomography (SPECT)," *Journal of the American Medical Association* 263 (1990): 561–64.

34. J. S. Krohmer, "Radiography and Fluoroscopy 1920 to the Present," *Radio-Graphics* 9 (1989): 1129–53.

35. J. G. Z. des Plantes, "Subtraction," *Fortschritte auf dem Gebiete der Röntgenstrahlen* 52 (1935): 69.

36. A. E. James, J. H. Anderson, and C. B. Higgins, *Digital Image Processing in Radiology* (Baltimore: Williams and Wilkins Company, 1985).

37. T. F. Meany, "Invasive Radiology," *Radio-Graphics* 9 (1989): 1181–88.

10. Further Advances with Computers, 1980s and 1990s

1. *Nobel Prize Winners: An H. W. Wilson Biographical Dictionary* (New York: H. W. Wilson Company, 1987), p. 797.

2. Ibid., p. 848.

3. I. L. Pykett et al., "Principles of Nuclear Magnetic Resonance Imaging," *Radiology* 143 (1982): 157–68.

4. *Nobel Prize Winners,* pp. 841, 102.

5. J. Mallard, "The Do's Have It," *British Journal of Radiology* 54 (1981): 831–49; Pykett et al., "Principles," pp. 157–68.

6. T. L. James and A. R. Margulis, "Historical Development of Biomedical Magnetic Resonance," *Biomedical Magnetic Resonance* 147 (1984): 1–3; R. Lenkinski, "Magnetic Resonance Spectroscopy, Basic Principles," *MRI Decisions* 3 (1989): 23–31.

7. C. B. Bratton, A. L. Hopkins, and J. W. Weinberg, "Nuclear Magnetic Resonance in Living Muscle," *Science* 147 (1965): 738–39; T. R. Ligon (thesis manuscript, Oklahoma State University, 1967); J. A. Jackson and W. H. Langham, "Whole Body NMR Spectrometer," *Review of Scientific Instruments* 39 (1968): 510–13.

8. R. Damadian, "Tumor Detection by Nuclear Magnetic Resonance," *Science* 171 (1971): 1151–53; I. D. Weisman et al., "Recognition of Cancer In Vivo by Nuclear Magnetic Resonance," *Science* 178 (1972): 1288–90; D. P. Hollis and L. A. Saryan, "A Nuclear Magnetic Resonance Study in Two Morris Hepatomas," *Johns Hopkins Medical Journal* 131 (1972): 441–44.

9. S. Kleinfeld, *A Machine Called Indomitable* (New York: Times Books, 1985).

10. P. Lauterbur, "Image Information by Induced Local Interactions: Examples Employing Nuclear Magnetic Resonance," *Nature* 242 (1973): 190–91.

11. P. Lauterbur, "Cancer Detection by Nuclear Magnetic Resonance Zeugmatography Imaging," *Cancer* 57 (1986): 1899–1904.

12. D. D. Stark and W. G. Bradley, *Magnetic Resonance Imaging* (St. Louis: C. V. Mosby Company, 1988).

13. James and Margulis, "Historical Development," p. 2.

14. W. R. Hendee, "Cross Sectional Medical Imaging," *Radio-Graphics* 9 (1989): 1155–80.

15. P. Sprawls, *Physical Principles of Medical Imaging* (Rockville, Md.: Aspen Publishers, 1987); H. S. Smith and F. N. Ranallo, *A Non-mathematical Approach to Basic MRI* (Madison, Wis.: Medical Physics Publishing Corp., 1989).

16. D. L. Miller et al., "Cardiovasular/Interventional Radiology," *Radiology* 190 (1994): 607.

17. P. A. Rinck, G. Nilsen, and O. Smevik, "Contrast Agents," *Medical Focus* 6 (1989): 11–16.

18. W. M. Angus, "A Commentary on the Development of Diagnostic Imaging Technology," *Radio-Graphics* 9 (1990): 1225–44; M. W. Weiner, "Magnetic Resonance Spectroscopy and Spectroscopic Imaging," *Administrative Radiology* 9 (1990): 32–40.

Epilogue

1. E. J. Ferris et al., "Percutaneous Angioscopy," *Radiology* 157 (1985): 319; A. Ganssen and H. Koening, "Status and Future Prospective of MR Tomography in Medical Diagnostics," *Electromedica* 54 (1986): 3.

2. T. Lücke, *Tagebücher und Aufzeichnungen von Leonardo da Vinci* (Berlin: Akad. Verlag, 1940).

3. G. Spiegler, "A Trip to Lennep, the Birthplace of Roentgen," *British Journal of Radiology* 40 (1967): 875.

4. A. B. Chain, "Reflections on the Future of Medicine and Research," as quoted in *Medical Tribune,* Sept., 1966.

5. G. Crile, *Intelligence, Power, and Personality* (New York: McGraw Hill, 1941).

6. "Education: Leaders of the 21st Century," *Time,* April 28, 1980, p. 81.

7. Jonathon Jacky, "Programmed for Disaster," *The Sciences* (New York Academy of Science), Sept.–Oct., 1989.

8. John von Neumann, *The Computer and the Brain* (New Haven: Yale University Press, 1974).

Index

Abdomen, noninvasive
visualization of, 113
ACTA. *See* Automated
computerized transverse axial
(ACTA) scanner
Adrenal glands, 113
Alexander, B., 81
Alexander the Great, 9, 11, 12, 28
Alexandria: as center of learning,
12–15, 17, 19–21, 133; decline
of, 21–23, 26; Galen in, 24;
siege of, 27; Ibn al-Nafis in, 29
Alwens, W., 66–67, 76
Ambrose, J., 109–10
Anaxagoras, 12, 15
Anesthesia: mandrake used as, 19;
Sicard's use of, 73
Aneurysms: Dos Santos's studies
of, 78; radiology for, 119;
Rowntree's studies of, 76;
Vesalius's diagnosis of, 47
Anger, H. O., 118
Angiography: Brooks's
contributions to, 77;
Castellanos's studies in, 81;
computerization of, 118; CT in,
125; Des Plantes's contributions
to, 81; Haschek's contributions
to, 65; Leonardo's experiments
as precursor of, 38; micro-
angiography, 99; Moniz's
contributions to, 78; and MRI,

127; Robb-Steinberg
contributions to, 82; and
uroselectan, 79
Animals: Aristotle's study of, 9;
Cannon's studies of, 67;
Dandy's studies of, 73; as
disease vectors, 4; early
dissections of, 1–2, 9, 24, 26;
Erasistratus's study of, 17, 25;
Forssmann's studies of, 79–80;
Franck-Alwens studies of,
66–67; Galen's study of, 24–26;
Graham-Cole studies of, 75;
Hevesy's studies of, 83–84;
Hooke's studies of, 52;
Hounsfield's studies of, 109;
Kinmouth's studies of, 102;
Leonardo's study of, 38;
Moniz's studies of, 77; and MRI
trials, 122–23; Schwann's
studies of, 53; Vesalius's study
of, 46
Aortography, 78–79
Archimedes, 15, 19, 23
Aristarchus, 15, 23
Aristotle, 8–9, 11–13, 16–17, 34,
36, 43–47
Arteries: Aristotle on, 9; Brooks's
studies of, 77; CT innovations
for, 125; Egyptians on, 2;
Erasistratus on, 18, 25; Fallo-
pius on, 49–50; Franck-Alwens

161

T. DOBY, M.D., F.A.C.R., is a member of the New York Academy of Sciences and previously was a staff member of the X-ray Department of Yale University. He is presently a director emeritus of the X-ray Department of Mercy Hospital in Portland, Maine. In addition to numerous scientific articles, he is the author of *Discoverers of Blood Circulation* and *Development of Angiography and Cardiovascular Catheterization.*

G. ALKER, M.D., was a professor and chair of the Radiology Department of the State University of New York at Buffalo. In addition to numerous scientific articles, he contributed to the book *Head Injury,* edited by L. Bakay, M.D., and F. E. Glasaver. He also published the detailed chapter (with S. Rudin and D. Bednarek) "Computed Tomography" in *The Encyclopedia of Medical Devices and Instrumentation* and was the associate editor of the leading specialty journal *Computerized Radiology.*